Endometriosis from Harm to Hope
A Chronic Illness Guide

CASEY BERNA, LCSW

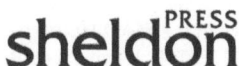

First published by Sheldon Press in 2026
An imprint of John Murray Press

1

Copyright © Casey Berna, LCSW 2026

The right of Casey Berna, LCSW to be identified as the Author of the Work has been asserted by her in accordance with the Copyright, Designs and Patents Act 1988.

The acknowledgments constitute an extension of this copyright page.

All rights reserved. No part of this publication may be reproduced, stored in a retrieval system, or transmitted, in any form or by any means without the prior written permission of the publisher, nor be otherwise circulated in any form of binding or cover other than that in which it is published and without a similar condition being imposed on the subsequent purchaser.

This book is for information or educational purposes only and is not intended to act as a substitute for medical advice or treatment. Any person with a condition requiring medical attention should consult a qualified medical practitioner or suitable therapist.

A CIP catalogue record for this title is available from the British Library

Trade Paperback ISBN 9781399822909
ebook ISBN 9781399822916

Typeset by KnowledgeWorks Global Ltd.

Printed and bound in Great Britain by Clays Ltd, Elcograf S.p.A.

John Murray Press policy is to use papers that are natural, renewable and recyclable products and made from wood grown in sustainable forests. The logging and manufacturing processes are expected to conform to the environmental regulations of the country of origin.

John Murray Press	Sheldon Press
Carmelite House	Hachette Book Group
50 Victoria Embankment	123 South Broad Street
London EC4Y 0DZ	Ste 2750
	Philadelphia, PA 19109, USA

www.sheldonpress.co.uk

John Murray Press, part of Hodder & Stoughton Limited
An Hachette UK company

The authorised representative in the EEA is Hachette Ireland, 8 Castlecourt Centre, Dublin 15, D15 XTP3, Ireland (email: info@hbgi.ie)

*This book is dedicated to my brave and resilient daughter.
May disease or illness never make you doubt your self-worth.
May you never mistake your lack of capacity for a lack of
competence. May you always believe your lived experiences.
May you never suffer fools who invalidate you.
May you always feel loved.*

Contents

1	What is Endometriosis?	1
2	Why is Endometriosis Uniquely Challenging to Treat?	17
3	Endometriosis: Sexual and Reproductive Health	33
4	It's Almost Never Just Endo: Common Comorbidities	65
5	Sick and Tired of Feeling Sick and Tired and Other Mental Health Impacts	91
6	From Harm to Hope	123

Appendix A: Endometriosis Treatment and Support Protocol for all Providers	185
Acknowledgments	189
Resources	191
Supporting Research	195
Index	207
About the author	211

1
What is Endometriosis?

My whole body felt like it was failing and no one could tell me why. My periods were excruciating, making it extremely difficult to get out of bed. It felt like there was a mob of gremlins in my pelvis with metal cleats on, doing a punishing, up-tempo jig in unison that left me swollen and hunched over for days.

Throughout the month, I depended on anti-diarrhea medicine to leave the house and when I did have a more solid bowel movement, it felt like it was covered in razor blades, tearing my rectum apart as it left my body. Often after bigger meals, I would vomit, as if my system was rejecting the work it would take to digest. Nausea persisted. Sleep eluded me as I was getting up a few times a night to urinate.

I also could feel my body ovulate, as if my ovaries were tearing apart with every cycle. Intercourse was so painful, yet my desire to overcome my struggle with infertility caused me to bear it, tears flowing down my eyes, the pain would linger for hours. The fatigue was breathtaking, impeding daily tasks and constantly making me crave bedtime, which came earlier and earlier.

Wearing pants was hard. Going more than ten minutes in a car was hard. Eating was hard. Breathing without pain was hard. Being social was hard. Working and being in school was hard. Standing was hard. Sitting was hard.

Existing was hard ... and no doctor could tell me why.
–Morgan, age 26

Despite its prevalence, many people have never even heard of endometriosis, and even some of the most educated and respected medical providers do not have a grasp on the devastation endometriosis can cause.

Endometriosis is a systemic, inflammatory disease that can impact nearly every organ system in the body. By definition, endometriosis is the presence of endometriotic lesions (or tissue) found in various locations *outside* of the uterus. These lesions are similar in nature to the tissue that lines the uterus, except endometriotic lesions create their own estrogen and stimulate the release of excess prostaglandins, often inciting an inflammatory response from our body's immune system. The inflammatory response is our body's way of trying to heal, yet the body is not able to eradicate the lesions. Pain, inflammation, organ dysfunction, fibrosis, and adhesions commonly develop wherever endometriosis exists and also contributes to systemic inflammation throughout the body.

Think about endometriosis as a thumbtack in your hand. That thumbtack does not belong and your body's natural immune response to this intruder is pain, inflammation, and swelling. The longer the thumbtack stays in your hand, the more it impacts the surrounding tissue, muscles and nerves in the hand, limiting the overall function of that hand. As your body tries to adapt to the thumbtack, your body will favor other parts to avoid the pain that comes with using the impacted hand. The mere presence of the thumbtack causes injury and an inflammatory response and as long as that thumbtack is there, the body is going to have something to say about it.

Now picture endometriosis as an unwelcome intruder located throughout your body. Endometriotic lesions can exist on the bladder, the bowels, the appendix, the diaphragm, as well as other organs. It can manifest as endometriomas on the ovaries, and even be found in the lungs or wrapped around the sciatic nerve. The longer endometriosis remains in our body, the more we are at risk for the endometriotic implants to deepen, new blood vessels feeding the disease to develop, more scar tissue and adhesions to form, more multifactorial pain to develop, including nerve pain, while organ dysfunction increases.

Endometriosis can be an excruciating and invasive disease that impacts 1 in 10 individuals assigned female at birth, and less commonly has been found in cisgender males. Millions of people suffer from endometriosis around the globe, but the majority of us wait many painful years for a diagnosis. At large, most providers and the medical community are not familiar with the proper definition of the disease nor the impact it can have on our body.

Like the majority of endometriosis patients that I see in my mental health practice, I too suffered with myriad painful and invasive symptoms before receiving any answers. I went from provider to provider, enduring many tests and ultrasounds, and always came away with more questions than answers. Even when I finally received an endometriosis diagnosis, the doctor who gave it to me didn't explain the magnitude of the disease nor how it can impact so many systems in my body.

Myths Dispelled: What Endometriosis is *Not*

For years, I experienced horrific endometriosis symptoms while also going through infertility and recurrent pregnancy loss. My doctor kept telling me that if only I could stay pregnant, my endometriosis would get better.

Time and time again we are fed myths about endometriosis, not only from well-meaning family and friends who are trying to be helpful, but also from healthcare providers who lack awareness of the disease. They make us feel like we are to blame for our continued pain and symptoms. And as a result, we leave waiting rooms feeling dismissed and invalidated, creating obstacles to diagnosis and treatment.

Endometriosis is *not* just a bad period. Too many providers still think of endometriosis as the lining of the uterus gone rogue. But pigeonholing endometriosis as only monster period cramps leads providers to ignore signs of endometriosis in those without a period. While endometriosis can cause painful periods, it is not just a menstrual disease. Endometriosis has been found in young patients before they even get their periods. Significant endometriosis has been found in postmenopausal patients. Endometriosis has also been found in females born without uteruses and those who have had their uterus removed.

Endometriosis is not just a reproductive disease. Unfortunately, our historically paternalistic and misogynistic society has often tied a woman's value to fertility, being a mother, and sexually pleasing her partner (often assumed male). As a result, endometriosis diagnosis and treatment has centered around our fertility and sexual health and ignored other crucial aspects of the disease. Those of us who have no interest in building a family are dismissed and told to come back when ready for family building or given the option of a hysterectomy.

While endometriosis can impact fertility and sexual health, it is far from the only thing. Endometriosis can also impact the ten other systems in the body including:

- the digestive system
- the urinary system
- the respiratory system
- the cardiovascular system
- the endocrine system
- the lymphatic system
- the nervous system
- the musculoskeletal system
- the immune system
- the integumentary system.

Endometriosis is *not* simply a hormone imbalance. If you have struggled with endometriosis, you have probably heard that maybe your hormones are just out of whack and that you have to just get them back on track. There are providers and wellness companies making millions from patients in pain looking for solutions to treat their endometriosis through "hormone balancing." While there are hormonal medical treatments which aim to alleviate symptoms, at this time, there are no hormonal-based treatments or therapies that shrink, cure or stop the growth of endometriosis—and definitely no supplements, elixirs, or cleansing regiments that cure endometriosis.

Endometriosis is *not* a curable disease. One of the hardest things about having endometriosis is that unfortunately, at this time, there is no cure. Pregnancy will not cure endometriosis. A hysterectomy (with or without ovary removal) will not cure endometriosis, as the disease by definition exists outside of the uterus. The lifelong treatment goal of endometriosis patients is to surgically excise as much endometriosis as possible, from all implicated organs, restore function to impacted areas, and continue with multidisciplinary care to support the body and reduce inflammation as much as possible.

When working with patients in my practice, this is one of the most difficult things to come to terms with. With support, patients work to grieve this loss and adapt to what it means to be an endometriosis patient.

Endometriosis is *not* just a white women's disease. I have witnessed the detrimental impact discriminatory bias has on endometriosis patients who are a part of the BIPOC and LGBTQIA+ communities. Endometriosis impacts people of all races and ethnicities. Endometriosis also impacts the transgender, nonbinary, and gender-expansive community assigned female at birth. Endometriosis on the rare occasion even impacts cisgender men.

Endometriosis is *not* caused by sexual trauma. If you have experienced sexual trauma and have endometriosis, you need more trauma-informed care and less obstacles to care. But patients can be further traumatized when medical providers and mental health providers blame their obvious endometriosis symptoms on their history of sexual trauma. People who have and have not experienced sexual trauma both get endometriosis. Those with histories of sexual trauma, who are navigating endometriosis, may benefit from extra support as they may experience added challenges, stressors, and pain due to their history of trauma.

Endometriosis is *not* "in the patient's head." If *only* endometriosis was truly like having a thumbtack in your hand! That is a health problem everyone would be able to recognize and treat! Unfortunately, due to misdiagnosis, delays in diagnosis, and a general lack of education and awareness, the continued symptoms we experience are often dismissed, true disease ignored, and we are sent for a psychiatric evaluation to address our *perceived* symptoms. We do not suffer because we are weak or have the wrong mindset. We suffer because we are sick and have a real disease inside of us that causes excruciating pain and fatigue. We suffer because at any given moment our organs may be stuck together and not functioning properly. While there have been a few, extremely rare, cases of brain endometriosis reported, the overwhelming majority of endometriosis is indeed not actually in our head!

Endometriosis is *not* something the patient has to get over and endure. Endometriosis is a painful disease that, for many of us, requires a lot of support and intervention. This is not something we can "grin and bear." The level of pain and intrusive symptoms that many of us have are not normal or sustainable. This is not something we can learn to live with without support managing and treating the symptoms.

Endometriosis is *not* the patient's fault. We do not have endometriosis because we are overweight or underweight. We do not have the disease because we aren't vegan or because we drink soda. It's not because we don't exercise or because we are stressed. We don't have endometriosis because we are sexually active, or because we had an abortion, or because we have been or haven't been on the birth control pill. It's not because we don't do yoga or take vitamins. Endometriosis is a chronic, painful, invasive and challenging disease that exists in the body, most likely due to our genetic disposition, although exact origins are still being explored. Patients who have first-degree relatives who have endometriosis are at an increased risk for having it.

Symptoms of Endometriosis

Over the span of ten years, I started developing seemingly unrelated symptoms that were painful, uncomfortable, inconvenient, and intrusive to my quality of life. I had horrible pain with my period and ovulation. My unpredictable, and at times, explosive, bowel movements made it hard to travel or go out to eat. I had to urinate all of the time. I was tired in a way that made it hard to function, and that no amount of sleep could cure. At 26 years old, I also was classified as infertile after trying, unsuccessfully, to get pregnant. Most of my providers chalked my symptoms up to stress and anxiety. Looking back, it was so obvious that I had endometriosis. When my clients come in with these symptoms, within minutes I suspect endometriosis and refer them to an endometriosis specialist and educational resources to further explore.

The most common symptoms associated with endometriosis are painful, and sometimes heavy periods, as well as general chronic pelvic pain outside of menstruation. Abdominal bloating and fatigue are also experienced by the vast majority of patients. Patients commonly report that their symptoms disrupt their quality of life, although we are expected to push through the pain.

Symptoms vary and in some cases, severe endometriosis has been found in patients who report being asymptomatic. Pain is not necessarily related with disease severity as even patients with a small amount of disease can have a great amount of pain. Symptoms may correlate to where endometriosis is in our body, although more clinical research needs to be done to support this.

Symptoms often associated with the reproductive system:

- painful periods
- painful ovulation
- painful intercourse/penetration
- pain with tampon insertion
- chronic pelvic pain
- infertility
- pregnancy loss
- ectopic pregnancy
- adverse birth outcomes/complications such as preterm labor.

Symptoms often associated with the digestive system:

- nausea
- diarrhea
- constipation
- painful bowel movements
- bloating.

Symptoms often associated with disease impacting the urinary system:

- frequent urination
- bladder pain
- lower back pain.

Symptoms often associated with disease impacting the respiratory system:

- chest pain
- rib pain
- lung collapses
- difficulty breathing
- coughing up blood.

Symptoms often associated with disease impacting the nervous system:

- leg pain
- hip pain
- neuropathy.

It's not uncommon for some patients to have these health issues as well:

- chronic fatigue
- migraines
- allergies
- other comorbidities, especially adenomyosis, female bladder pain syndrome, appendicitis, cholecystectomy, and immune-related disorders.

Endometriosis Throughout the Lifespan

My pain started on the first day of my period when I was just 12 years old. Looking back, I had weird food allergies, headaches and other symptoms long before even getting my period. I now wonder if that was endometriosis related.

Right before my 14th birthday, I finally went to the gynecologist to talk about my painful menstrual bleeding, my nausea, my right-sided pain, especially in the middle of my cycle, my fatigue and my constipation. Going to school was getting harder, especially on days when I had my period. I was losing weight as the pain and nausea throughout the month made it difficult to eat. My mom came with me to the appointment. She had many surgeries for endometriosis and we were pretty sure it was behind the symptoms I was having. The gynecologist listened to my symptoms and offered birth control. We asked about endometriosis, and she told us teens do not get endometriosis.

After a year of trying different birth control pills, the pain and other symptoms just got worse. We traveled out of state to see an endometriosis specialist who, through surgical excision of the disease, diagnosed me officially with endometriosis. It was throughout my entire pelvis, on my colon, my bladder, my rectum, and was causing my appendix, which had to be removed, to stretch and adhere to other organs. My ovaries were also stuck to the back of my pelvic sidewall.

–Hailey, age 16

I often wonder what would have happened if someone had identified my symptoms as endometriosis back when I was a teenager. How would that have changed my experience in college as I struggled to work, go to class, and do my social work internships? How would it have helped my fertility and family building if I had had that information? Those of us who go ten, twenty years, and sometimes even longer without a diagnosis, endure more years of gaslighting and physical harm. It seems there is only a slim window in which endometriosis is on the radar of providers, even though it exists within our bodies at every stage of life.

Many, otherwise reliable, medical websites state that endometriosis is most common for those of childbearing age, particularly those in their thirties and forties. Often, they'll include a remark about how it can impact fertility. Many in the medical community hold this same belief.

The truth is that endometriosis has been found in fetuses, as early as 25 weeks gestation. Endometriosis has been found in newborns. One case study highlighted a six-year-old who was surgically diagnosed with an ovarian endometrioma, a cystic lesion that stems from the disease process of endometriosis, well before menstruation began. There have been other pediatric cases reported as well. It is not uncommon for endometriosis patients to have experienced our first symptoms before the age of 15.

The reality is that teens have endometriosis and suffer tremendously because of the disease. According to The American College of Obstetricians and Gynecologists (ACOG) Committee Opinion on Dysmenorrhea and Endometriosis in the Adolescent, at least *two thirds* of adolescents born female with chronic pelvic pain, who are unresponsive to hormonal therapies and NSAIDs, will be diagnosed with endometriosis at the time of diagnostic laparoscopy. Yet, even with this data, adolescents who come to their provider in agonizing pain are often told that teens do not get diagnosed with endometriosis. Our abnormal pain is normalized and we get prescribed birth control to try to manage symptoms.

The struggle to get care and a diagnosis only continues. In our twenties, we see our provider and list chronic pelvic pain and other obvious endometriosis symptoms. And, instead of investigating further, they prescribe us hormonal treatments or tell us we should think about having a baby sooner rather than later to fix our pain. It doesn't even matter if having a child is part of our current life plan or if we are even in a relationship with a partner, never mind one with shared intentions to have a family.

In our thirties and forties, providers more readily recognize endometriosis *if* we are white and struggling with infertility. But by then, the disease has been thriving in our bodies for decades. By this time, we often are experiencing a whole host of symptoms, impacting many systems in our body, and have multiple providers throughout different areas of medicine struggling to put the whole picture together. Here's an example of a list of providers and their (very different) goals for dealing with the same disease:

Provider(s)	*Goal*
Reproductive endocrinologists	Get us pregnant or freeze our eggs for future pregnancies.
Gastroenterologists	Figure out why our bowels are causing pain and not functioning properly
Urologists	Figure out why our bladders are causing pain and not functioning properly
Immunologists	Find source of our chronic fatigue
Pulmonologist	Find source of our diaphragmatic pain and shortness of breath
Orthopedist	Find source of our sciatic or hip pain

An official endometriosis diagnosis often still remains elusive for many of us during this time as providers do not recognize these symptoms as potential endometriosis.

Once providers are convinced we are done with family building, they recommend a hysterectomy, which they are taught is a definitive treatment, even though it doesn't address endometriosis, a disease defined as *outside* of the uterus. If we have had a hysterectomy, or are in menopause, a potential endometriosis diagnosis falls off the radar of providers completely. We are back to square one in terms of getting providers to believe that endometriosis can be causing our pain and symptoms. Most providers, associating endometriosis with period pain, believe that once a patient's period is gone, so is the endometriosis. But when we still have continued bladder, bowel, and sciatic endometriosis symptoms, they attribute these to other things.

Misdiagnosis and the Challenges of Diagnosis

> My hairstylist is the one who helped diagnose me with endometriosis and connect me to needed treatment. I had been to a half-dozen OB/GYNs in my city over the span of a decade, and they kept diagnosing me with chronic pelvic pain. After years of birth control and pelvic floor therapy, my symptoms were just getting worse. Ultrasound after ultrasound showed nothing. I kept asking what they thought the source of the pain was and they didn't have an answer.
>
> After a particularly frustrating doctor's appointment, I started crying during my hair appointment and told my hairstylist about my health struggles. He immediately asked if I knew about endometriosis and connected me with a local expert that another client of his went to. A few months later, I was getting the treatment I needed and had an official diagnosis. My hairstylist, in ten minutes, helped me in a way that doctors couldn't do over ten years.
>
> –Jordan, age 36

Diagnosis is elusive for many of us for a multitude of reasons. Shame and stigma surrounding talking about reproductive health challenges and uncomfortable symptoms can make us delay reporting our symptoms to providers. The lack of awareness of the disease, normalization of pain, medical racism and paternalism throughout the medical industrial complex, and limited access to expert medical care are just some of the many systemic challenges that we face.

We often do not look sick to providers, so endometriosis is often considered an invisible disease. In a 2017 newsletter to OB/GYNs, ACOG's then president, Tom Gellhaus MD, shared disturbing, yet unsurprising statistics: "Up to 63% of general practitioners feel uncomfortable diagnosing and treating patients with endometriosis. And as many as half are unfamiliar with the three main symptoms of the disease." One survey recently showed that it can take almost four years from onset of symptoms for patients to share what they are experiencing with their provider, then it can take an average of six more years before getting a diagnosis. For the average patient, that is a decade of suffering without answers or intervention.

By the time I was 23 years old, years before I was diagnosed with endometriosis, I had endured multiple vaginal ultrasounds, MRIs, CT scans, Upper Gastrointestinal Series, Lower Gastrointestinal Series, multiple colonoscopies, and an appendectomy for what was considered "borderline appendicitis." During that time not one provider mentioned even the possibility of endometriosis, and it did not show up on any of those tests. My experience is not unique and I hear similar stories from other patients daily.

Our biggest challenge is that currently the only way to get an official endometriosis diagnosis is through surgical biopsy and pathological confirmation of disease during laparoscopic surgery. Laparoscopic surgery is a minimally invasive surgical technique utilizing a laparoscope, which is a camera that is inserted in the abdomen through a small incision. During laparoscopic surgery other small incisions are made for surgical tools used to remove disease or impacted organs.

Surgical Excision and Pathological Confirmation

If providers had X-ray vision and could see the damage and horrors that endometriosis can cause in our bodies, we would access treatment far more easily. It seems unbelievable, but the only way to get true confirmation of the disease is to have a surgeon go in, cut out a sample of suspected endometriosis and then send it to pathology for confirmation.

This depends on the provider doing the surgery and their knowledge of the different presentations and locations of the disease in your body, and their skills to excise the disease in those places. There have been some patients who have had surgery with one provider, and were told there was no endometriosis to be found, only to get a diagnostic confirmation after going to a more educated and skilled surgeon who then found the disease.

Surgery, and recovery from surgery, requires a lot of resources and is not accessible to all patients. The idea of surgery can also be overwhelming for some. Though, the benefits of getting diagnosed in this way, especially by a recommended endometriosis excision expert, is that disease, adhesions, and scar tissue can be excised at the same time and organ function can be restored.

Methods for a Suspected Diagnosis

Getting a suspected diagnosis for endometriosis, can empower you to learn more about the disease so you can get needed support. If you have been suffering for years, with no answers, naming what could be making you sick and having a potential diagnosis can bring hope and lessen anxiety. The following are ways that you might learn that you potentially have endometriosis:

Patient History

You can give yourself a suspected diagnosis by researching your symptoms online, relating to them and learning more about the disease. Through taking a thorough medical history, your provider (or hairstylist!) can suspect endometriosis. You can relay this information in ten minutes or less. The challenge then becomes having a knowledgeable, or at the very least an open-minded provider, that will listen to these symptoms and provide a referral to an expert in endometriosis care.

Imaging

Certain endometriosis centers of care have modernized imaging machines, as well as dedicated and educated radiologists and providers who know how to recognize endometriosis on medical imaging, including ultrasounds, MRIs, and CT scans. Some in the endometriosis community have made a big push to accept that endometriosis can be seen and diagnosed through imaging alone, but sadly that is not something all patients have access to at this time.

Receiving the dreaded "unremarkable," "typical," or "normal" scans, can feel discouraging when in reality, there is nothing normal or typical about your pain and symptoms. Patients with normal scans are told by well-meaning providers that there is nothing wrong with them, and the delay in diagnosis and needed treatment continues. It is important to note that a negative imaging result does not exclude endometriosis.

Ultrasounds can often see and identify ovarian endometriomas, cystic lesions on the ovary. Only people with endometriosis get endometriomas, so it is important to assess whether or not those with endometriomas have signs and symptoms of disease elsewhere. Some estimate that up to 50% of people with deeply infiltrating endometriosis have endometriomas. Also, research shows that up to 30% of people with endometriosis have bowel involvement. Often, endometriomas are diagnosed or treated without acknowledging an endometriosis diagnosis or the potential for further disease involvement, leading again to a delay in diagnosis and intervention.

Sometimes scans show hydronephrosis of the kidneys or swelling of the kidneys. This can be a sign of endometriosis on the ureters, which can impact the flow of urine. If you have ureteral endometriosis, you are at risk for silent kidney loss, which can happen when disease is left untreated.

An MRI might reveal rectal nodules, depending on their size. However, note that the lack of nodules does not rule out bowel endometriosis.

Lung collapse or pneumothorax, especially during the time of menstruation, can indicate thoracic endometriosis. A chest X-ray or a CT scan can help diagnose a pneumothorax.

Blood Tests

While many companies are developing blood tests for endometriosis markers, none of these tests are definitive. You may be encouraged to partake in hormone therapies to treat your "possible endometriosis," based on the results of these tests alone. It's important to note that some of the makers of the blood tests also have financial ties to the same hormone therapies recommended. Consulting with multidisciplinary endometriosis specialists will give you greater insights into potential disease and treatments.

Medical Therapy

Some providers try to diagnose you by giving you hormonal-based medical treatments and waiting for a difference in your symptoms. Providers feel that if symptoms are relieved, then endometriosis can be suspected. Without surgical confirmation of the disease, it is impossible to be sure whether you have endometriosis, or other diagnoses that can cause similar symptoms such as adenomyosis, or fibroids. Hormonal medical therapy may reduce symptoms for some, but it doesn't diagnose or cure the disease, and the disease can still cause harm.

Most patient advocates and expert multidisciplinary providers in the endometriosis community are calling for a culture of referral for suspected endometriosis patients. When you have a suspected endometriosis diagnosis and see an expert in care, they are able to give you informed consent, helping you understand the benefit and challenges to all treatment options and provide more tools and multidisciplinary support as you learn to navigate this challenging disease.

2
Why is Endometriosis Uniquely Challenging to Treat?

In the span of five years, I had multiple pelvic surgeries with my local OB/GYN to try to get relief from my endometriosis. I also had been on half a dozen different types of hormonal medication, to include one that made me feel like I was in menopause. Nothing gave me more than short-term relief.

Slowly, my life started to fall apart. I had to drop out of law school and I could barely keep my part-time job as a paralegal. My doctor was recommending a hysterectomy, but at 30 years old, I wasn't ready for that. Through an online community I found a surgeon who focused on endometriosis. After a five hour surgery, I learned that my uterus was healthy, but I had significant, deeply infiltrating endometriosis on my bowels that my local doctors kept missing. I also had a lot of adhesions and scar tissue from my previous surgeries.

While removing so much disease from my bowels helped, I also learned that I needed other complementary care to help me heal. Taking care of my body sometimes feels like a full-time job, but I finally feel like I am starting to live my life again.

–Joey, age 32

Multidisciplinary Treatment

Endometriosis is a complex disease that can be very challenging to treat. Many of the top providers and patient advocates agree that treating endometriosis takes a multidisciplinary approach that can include medical management and surgical excision along with other multidisciplinary care.

Medical management is one approach used to try to reduce the symptoms of endometriosis. The most common medications prescribed to patients by the majority of OB/GYNs are:

- NSAIDS
- combined hormonal contraceptives

- progesterone and progestins
- GnRH agonists and GnRH antagonists.

NSAIDs

NSAIDS are nonsteroidal anti-inflammatory drugs. They are usually the first line of treatment for patients, as they can decrease pain and inflammation.

Benefits of NSAIDs:

- provides some relief from symptoms
- accessible
- affordable.

Drawbacks of NSAIDs:

- does not stop the progression of the disease or shrink existing lesions
- usually not enough to fully manage symptoms
- in high doses, causes gastrointestinal ulcers.

Combined Hormonal Contraceptives

Often, endometriosis excision experts and the majority of OB/GYNs both recommend combined hormonal contraceptives in the form of the pill, transdermal patch or vaginal ring. These suppress ovulation and menstruation and can reduce symptoms.

Benefits of hormonal contraceptives:

- may provide some relief from symptoms
- accessible
- affordable
- tolerable for long-term.

Drawbacks of hormonal contraceptives:

- does not stop the progression of the disease or shrink existing lesions
- side effects such as nausea, vomiting, breast tenderness, acne, weight gain and depression.

Progesterone and Progestins

Endometriosis excision experts and the majority of OB/GYNs alike recommend progesterone and progestins to reduce symptoms and improve menstrual pain. These medications are available in different forms including, oral, injectable, transdermal patches, vaginal rings, intrauterine devices, and subcutaneous implants.

Benefits of progesterone and progestin:

- may provide some relief from symptoms
- accessible
- affordable
- most forms tolerable for long-term.

Drawbacks of progesterone and progestin:

- does not stop the progression of the disease or shrink existing lesions
- side effects such as acne, mood changes, and weight gain
- irregular bleeding with intrauterine devices, especially at the start
- injectable contraceptive medroxyprogesterone acetate may increase risk of benign brain tumors with long-term use.

GnRH Agonists

GnRH agonists put you in a menopause-like state, and your local provider might recommend them after combined hormonal contraceptives, and progesterone-based medications stop reducing your symptoms. But be aware, GnRH agonists have not been proven to be more effective at treating endometriosis symptoms when compared to combined oral contraceptives, and progesterone-based medications.

However, patients report significant, sometimes intolerable, side effects with these medications and, for some, these symptoms can last even after stopping the medication. "Add-back" therapy is highly recommended to try to reduce side effects of the medication.

Benefits of GnRH agonists:

- may provide some relief from symptoms.

Drawbacks of GnRH agonists:

- only recommended for six months at a time
- does not stop the progression of the disease or shrink existing lesions
- not affordable for all
- significant side effects:
  - night sweats
  - vaginal dryness
  - mood changes
  - sleep disturbances
  - substantial reduction in bone mineral density that could increase risk of osteoporosis.

GnRH Antagonists

GnRH antagonists are another tool used by the majority of OB/GYNs to help treat the pain and symptoms of endometriosis. This class of drugs have slightly more tolerable side effects when compared to GnRh agonists, but if you can get pregnant, you'll need to take an oral contraceptive because of the risks and unfavorable outcomes the drug would cause to you and the fetus. Patients are encouraged to take "add-back" therapy to try to minimize serious long-term side effects, especially when taken at a higher dose.

More research needs to be done to see if these drugs are safe for long-term use and more effective for symptom reduction than combined hormonal contraceptives and progesterone, as GnRH antagonists are more expensive and patients report that side effects are more intolerable.

Benefits of GnRH antagonists:

- may provide some relief from symptoms
- slightly more tolerable side effects compared to GnRH agonists
- lower daily dosage than GnRH agonists.

Drawbacks of GnRH antagonists:

- does not stop the progression of the disease or shrink existing lesions
- not affordable for all
- significant side effects.

Surgical Treatment

After all other causes of infertility were ruled out, my reproductive endocrinologist suggested it may be endometriosis and scheduled my first surgery. After a 40-minute operation, he assured me I just had a little bit of endometriosis and that my fertility and quality of life was back on track. For the next few years his main focus was trying to get me pregnant through fertility treatments. Endometriosis would go on to invade my bladder wall, cause hydronephrosis in both kidneys, deeply infiltrate my bowels, and even impact my breathing due to creating scar tissue on my diaphragm. I know my experience reflects that of others in the community.

Surgical treatment for endometriosis is an important tool for relieving symptoms, along with restoring organ function and improving fertility. Endometriosis excision specialists and the majority of OB/GYNs often have a different approach to surgically treating endometriosis.

Expert Endometriosis Surgeon

This type of surgeon will systematically excise all of the endometriosis that they see. They often command a surgical team which may include a general surgeon, a colorectal surgeon, a urologist and sometimes even a cardiothoracic surgeon, depending on where endometriosis is suspected.

Over the course of a couple of hours, the surgeon will:

- restore your anatomy
- remove adhesions, scar tissue, and fibrosis
- cut out any endometriotic lesions, leaving a clear margin
- remove deeply infiltrating disease
- repair holes in any organs that are impacted, such as the bladder or diaphragm.

For deeply infiltrating endometriosis impacting the bowel, the surgeon will shave off the disease. For disease that has invaded the bowel wall, they will do a bowel resection. They will also check your appendix and gallbladder to make sure they are healthy and not impacted by endometriosis. Diseased organs will be removed.

It is highly unusual for an experienced excision surgeon to feel like disease is too risky to remove. If you are concerned about fertility, they will treat your reproductive organs with extreme care and check your fallopian tubes to assess risk for an ectopic pregnancy. They'll also check the inside of your bladder wall for inflammation, which can be another pelvic pain generator, and your uterus for adenomyosis.

The entire surgery will be recorded, and the team will take pictures for reference. They'll write up a post-operative report and a pathology report, which you'll be able to access later, along with the pictures. Meanwhile, the surgeon will send many tissue samples to pathology to get an official diagnosis. While it is not guaranteed that all disease will be removed, you'll often have better long-term relief rates with excision surgery and a lower rate of recurrence.

OB/GYNs

The majority of OB/GYNs cauterize or burn the surface of the endometriotic lesions, called the ablation technique. This technique only burns the surface of the disease, which means the bulk of the disease will still remain in place after surgery.

Most OB/GYNs perform surgeries that last under an hour and only focus on the reproductive organs, again leaving the majority of the disease in place. If the provider is not familiar with all of the presentations of the disease, they will likely leave endometriosis. Teenagers are especially at risk for this scenario because their disease can appear differently than someone in their thirties.

Not all providers take pictures during surgery or send samples to pathology. And because the disease is vaporized, there aren't any tissue samples to send to get tested for disease confirmation.

This type of surgery is often more easily covered by insurance and more accessible, but you can end up in more pain because of missed disease and the formation of more adhesions and scar tissue due to cauterization of tissue. Moreover, your average OB/GYN doesn't usually operate with a team and is not trained or experienced in removing extensive, deeply infiltrating endometriosis, so you are at risk of being told your disease is "too risky" to remove.

There is no cure for endometriosis and it is often seen as a chronic and progressive disease. Medical management by nature can only help reduce your symptoms while you are taking the medications. Even in the hands of the best endometriosis excision surgeon, you still need further therapeutic support to thrive. It takes a team to help heal the damage endometriosis causes.

Pelvic Floor Therapists

Endometriosis has a profound impact on the body over time and can cause dysfunction in the pelvic floor. Therefore, pelvic floor therapists are an important part of the multidisciplinary team.

Pelvic floor therapy can help:

- increase your mobility
- reduce your pain and inflammation
- ease difficulty urinating
- reduce difficulty having bowel movements
- make sex less painful
- lessen pain with movement.

Chronic pain can cause trauma to the muscles, ligaments, nerves, and fascia of the pelvis and abdominal wall. Even when the disease is removed, the body and the brain have to relearn how to function in a healthy way. Through stretches, breathing, and manual techniques, pelvic floor therapy can strengthen the pelvic floor while also allowing it to relax.

Other Providers to Consider

Mental health practitioners, pain management specialists, acupuncturists, nutritionists, and functional medicine practitioners are just some of the other professionals who are wonderful partners in multidisciplinary care for endometriosis.

Systemic Challenges to Endometriosis Treatment and the Harm They Cause

> I started my menstrual cycle when I was nine years old and it was heavy and painful. My mom, who didn't talk much about periods, told me that it was normal and how all the women in my family have the same thing. I knew fibroids were common in my family and in the African American community, but I had no idea if I was too young to have them and if fibroids were causing my pain.
>
> In high school, I had to go to the emergency room because the pain right before my period got so bad I passed out. The doctors there thought I was pregnant or had an STI, even though I told them I never had sex before. They wouldn't listen to me. When those tests came back negative and the scans and ultrasounds showed nothing, they started treating me like I was just looking for drugs. I had never taken anything other than tylenol in my life. They told me my pain wasn't that bad and there wasn't anything they could do. I left without any answers.
>
> It would be another six years of suffering before I would get an endometriosis diagnosis and finally learn why I was in so much pain.
> –Imani, age 20

There is no doubt in my mind that endometriosis is a social justice issue. Our physical and mental suffering exists at the systemic intersection of ignorance, paternalism, misogyny, racism, profits over patients, and an abysmal void of healthy equity. Over the decades, patient advocates have chipped away at these injustices, often at a cost to their own physical and mental health. Their hard work has moved the needle towards more awareness, more research funds, and better protections for patients. Yet, at this moment, those actually in charge of our well-being are still causing harm and those with power to change the systems that hurt us are failing to do so.

Uneducated and Unaware Providers

Estimates show that approximately 190 million people worldwide suffer with endometriosis. But despite the prevalence of the disease, many healthcare providers do not learn much about it in medical school. Even the majority of OB/GYNs do not have adequate training on endometriosis, including the main symptoms of the disease, the different systems of the body it impacts, or the varied presentations of the disease during surgery. The majority of OB/GYNs also do not have the same expertise that endometriosis specialists have in terms of treating the disease. Providers outside of gynecological care often have even less information about endometriosis.

This lack of awareness and education creates suffering, causing us physical harm as it leads to a delay in diagnosis and misdiagnosis, prolonging needed multidisciplinary treatment and support for this incredibly painful and invasive disease. When left undiagnosed and untreated, our pain, adhesions, scar tissue, and organ dysfucntion worsen, which significantly lowers quality of life and can also impact our fertility.

The emotional damage unaware and uneducated medical providers cause us can be just as harmful as the physical. Our symptoms are often dismissed or normalized. When treatments fail to make us feel better, some providers take their frustration out on us, even blame us for our continued pain. We are made to feel that we have failed treatments, even though research shows the majority of the treatments offered by the majority of OB/GYNs are known to fail endometriosis patients long term. The lack of awareness and education on the part of the provider can cause them to gaslight us into making us believe we are healthy or cured, even though we may still feel very ill and still have disease. When we spend years being treated this way, it profoundly impacts our mental health.

Endometriosis isn't a Gynecological Subspeciality

Gynecologic oncology, reproductive medicine, and maternal fetal medicine are just some of the subspecialties of gynecology. The medical community has deemed these issues important and complex enough to require further training. An average OB/GYN may screen for ovarian cancer, but they would never *treat* ovarian cancer. That patient would be referred immediately to a gynecological oncologist, who spends all of their time treating patients with cancer. They look at the latest research or even do research themselves. They attend conferences on gynecological cancer. They spend all day, every day treating cancer patients and have treated the most simple cases to the most complex. Gynecological oncologists are not monitoring pregnancies or delivering babies. They know the most about gynecologic cancers, therefore patients have better outcomes when going to see them.

Endometriosis is a disease so complex, so invasive, and so far-reaching, that it seems that it would be an obvious choice to put our well-being in the hands of specialists who spend the vast majority of their time treating endometriosis, researching endometriosis, and attending endometriosis conferences. But, there is currently not a subspecialty in endometriosis care, and the average OB/GYN is directed and empowered to treat endometriosis without referral to an expert in care.

In the US, gynecological providers rely on the ACOG's Management of Endometriosis Practice Bulletin for guidance on how to diagnose and treat endometriosis. These standards of care, that were originally written back in 2010, are not written by multidisciplinary endometriosis specialists, nor do they have the input of patient advocates. Most in the endometriosis community find these standards of care incomplete and harmful. In 2017, patient advocates and multidisciplinary providers petitioned the ACOG to update these standards of care, with the input of the community. Patients from all over the world also signed the petition, as the challenges that patients have in the United States also reflect the state of care in other countries around the world.

Even before the petition, advocates have long asked for updates to the standards of care, the creation of an endometriosis subspecialty, and a broader culture of referral. The lack of awareness and acceptance of the complexity of the disease often traps us on a merry-go-round of inadequate treatments and repeated surgeries, where the majority of the disease is left by providers whose treatment plans are supported by the current standards of care. The lack of recognition of endometriosis as a subspecialty also makes it easy for insurance companies to deny us access to expert providers when there is a closer OB/GYN who they feel is equipped to do the surgery.

While endometriosis is technically benign, when left untreated, the pain and dysfunction impacts every aspect of our lives causing great physical and emotional harm.

- How is it ethical to not refer endometriosis patients to an expert multidisciplinary team?
- How can the medical community allow providers who are not trained to identify all presentations of the disease, find disease in locations throughout the body, and fully excise the disease, operate on patients?
- Why is endometriosis seen as less deserving of a subspeciality than fertility or maternal fetal health?

These are questions patient advocates and leaders in multidisciplinary care have been asking for decades.

Accessibility

Ideally, there would be a dedicated multidisciplinary endometriosis center of care for every town and city. These centers would have an expert excision surgeon, mental health provider, pelvic floor therapist, as well as other multidisciplinary providers that specialize in the disease. Many cancer centers have adapted this model as it leads to better patient outcomes.

Unfortunately, many of us have to travel out of our city and sometimes even out of our home country to receive the care we need. This is often logistically impossible for some, adding expenses that are insurmountable. For example, those that live in rural areas often have to travel hours just to see a family medicine provider, never mind an endometriosis specialist. Some who live close to hospitals in economically challenged areas feel like they get better care if they travel to farther hospitals that have more resources, especially when going to the emergency department. These patients also have an incredibly difficult time accessing quality endometriosis care.

Over the years, many gynecological surgeons have advocated that they do not get adequately reimbursed for the surgeries they perform which causes challenges in covering the costs of providing the surgery. Surgeons performing procedures specific to those assigned female at birth have historically been reimbursed less than those performing comparable procedures on males. In the US, OB/GYNs who perform a 40-minute endometriosis ablation surgery, where the majority of the disease is often left untouched, get reimbursed the same amount as an expert excision surgeon who spends hours meticulously excising the disease. Some excision surgeons have left their positions at their hospital due to the pressure from administrators to perform the surgery as quickly as their OB/GYN counterparts to lessen costs. Because of this, some endometriosis providers have made the choice to operate out of network, which places a huge financial burden on us. Other multidisciplinary providers such as pelvic floor therapists, have also found it difficult to work with insurance companies as they don't feel compensated for their time and expertise.

For even the most privileged patients with access to the most resources, managing endometriosis is financially draining. For those who are uninsured, access to care feels impossible and they are left with little to no options. In the endometriosis community we often don't talk about those suffering who are unhoused, those who are incarcerated, those who are living in a refugee camp or a war-torn community, those without access to running water or who are food insecure. There are endometriosis patients who are suffering who may not even have access to over-the-counter pain medicine or menstrual products, never mind an expert multidisciplinary team.

Paternalism, Misogyny, Racism, Homophobia, Transphobia, and Cultural Incompetence

There is a popular meme that some medical providers have shared on the internet that states, "Please don't confuse your google search with my medical degree." Despite the fact that we are the consumers and are paying the medical providers for their time and care, we often feel an uneven power dynamic between ourselves and our providers. Because as endometriosis patients, we have been historically unsatisfied with the care we receive from providers, we are left to do our own research and advocate for our own care. Patient advocacy can be sometimes met with dismissal or even contempt from providers, instead of an open mind.

Both male and female providers can have internalized misogyny towards patients. Providers often see women as "baby makers" and value our fertility over quality of life. Providers blame our continued pain and health struggles on our weight, diet, exercise, or stress level. Providers have historically dismissed, ignored, and normalized our pain, calling us hysterical.

One also has to wonder if systemic paternalism and misogyny in the medical industrial complex also contributes to the failure to update standards of care for endometriosis, the failure to create a culture of referral and subspeciality for endometriosis, as well as the failure to adequately reimburse gynecological surgeons for the complex surgeries they perform. If millions of cisgender males were struggling with endometriosis and the infertility, sexual dysfunction, organ dysfunction and reduced quality of life it causes, would then patients be heard and changes made?

Black, Indigenous, and People of Color (BIPOC) have more obstacles to care than most in the endometriosis community. Systemic racism throughout the medical industrial complex, and implicit and explicit bias of providers and associated stigma harms patients. Research has shown that providers have beliefs rooted in racism that Black people have a higher pain tolerance which leads to the dismissal or undertreatment of pain. Black women and Latina women are more likely to experience delays in diagnosis, interrupted care, and also struggle more than white women to get evaluated for infertility. They are even pushed towards different treatment options: Black and Latina women are more likely to be given a hysterectomy than white women. The medical exploitation and torture of Black women throughout the history of modern medicine, combined with the continued medical racism that patients face today, also has caused a transgenerational trauma and mistrust of providers and the medical system in its entirety, leading to a delay in patients seeking treatment.

The thoughtlessness, and even prejudice of providers and practices can create an added risk of stress and trauma for the LGBTQIA+ community. When a provider doesn't use a patient's preferred pronoun, or even leave a space to ask for it on intake papers, that can contribute to a patient feeling unsafe. When medical staff attending to the patient show prejudice towards a patient and their partner, an environment that should be caring and validating can feel hostile and dangerous. Assumptions made by providers regarding the reproductive and family building choices of patients can make those struggling with endometriosis feel dismissed and invalidated. The lack of gender-neutral language on endometriosis websites, in support groups and in care settings, the lack of representation of LGBTQIA+ individuals in pamphlets about the disease or in stories shared, and the lack of research on how to care for transgender patients all contribute to the further isolation of patients and hesitancy to seek treatment.

Lack of Societal Understanding of Endometriosis and Stigma Surrounding Reproductive Health

When an elderly neighbor has the flu, the community knows how to come together to help. Some folks may drop off soup or offer to go grocery shopping. Family members will call to check in to see how that person is doing. If your coworker's wife has cancer, there may be a meal train or a fundraiser to help with expenses.

We often face challenges finding that same level of support. One reason is that endometriosis is not a well-known disease, despite the fact that millions of people suffer from it. That is partly because there is a stigma associated with openly talking about periods and reproductive health in general. Symptoms such as painful sex, diarrhea, heavy bleeding, and infertility can be hard for patients to talk about due to their invasive and sensitive nature. The lack of awareness and empathy for the disease leads to a lack of structural support. Time off for school or employment is given more easily for other health struggles. Even disability benefits are given to other illnesses more readily than endometriosis. This all puts added stress and pressure on us and can make us feel even more isolated and less supported.

Laws that Interfere with Medical Advice or Needed Treatments

Currently, throughout the US and also in many other parts of the world, politicians are making laws that are causing us more suffering. IVF and other fertility treatments, lifesaving medicine to treat ectopic pregnancies, access to birth control and other hormonal treatments, and treatment for pregnancy loss are just some of the medical care that has been questioned by politicians who have made attempts to ban them. Politicians have felt empowered to try to limit the autonomy we have over our own bodies and have inserted themselves in the provider-patient relationship.

Endometriosis can cause infertility and many of us rely on IVF and other fertility treatments to try to build our families. For younger people with endometriosis, egg freezing is a great way to try to preserve fertility. We are at greater risk for ectopic pregnancies, which require the termination of the pregnancy to save the fertility and life of the patient. Hormonal medical treatments such as the birth control pill or IUDs are prescribed to try to help reduce symptoms. Miscarriages can be incredibly painful for us, and drugs to help this process along are crucial to lessen physical and emotional suffering. Making access to this care harder causes us additional trauma during an already traumatic time.

3
Endometriosis
Sexual and Reproductive Health

I feel like every answer from my OB/GYN for my reproductive health struggles has always been to have a glass of wine and relax. Painful sex? Have a glass of wine! Trouble getting pregnant? Apparently, I work too much and need to take a vacation and have a glass of wine—it will happen! Frustrated, I eventually stopped bringing these issues up. We are now in the adoption process, and my OB/GYN is more convinced than ever that I am going to get pregnant, because in his experience, that always happens. Recently, I have been having a lot of health issues, which I honestly thought was stress from our recent move and the adoption process. But after having intense right-sided pain, which led to an emergency appendectomy, it turns out that I have a pelvis full of endometriosis. I am now waiting to see an endometriosis specialist and my guess is that all the wine in France would not cure this disease or its symptoms.

–Joy, age 34

Patriarchy in Women's Health

There are so many conflicting thoughts and messages about sexuality and reproductive health in our society. Most of our experiences as endometriosis patients exist at the intersection of these conflicting messages from society, our providers, and our family and friends, leaving us to feel alone and isolated.

Patriarchal views are deeply embedded in our society when it comes to sexuality and reproductive health. Throughout history, our value has often been placed in our body's ability to be a vessel for men's sexual pleasure and growing babies. Prescribing a glass of wine to a patient who is having pain with intercourse centers the needs of the patient's partner, as essentially it means just numbing the patient enough to allow intercourse to happen, not figuring out why it is painful or considering the harm of having sex while intoxicated.

When we come to our providers about our pain and discomfort linked to suspected endometriosis, sometimes they tell us to just go on birth control. They tell us we should address these issues when we are ready to have babies, clearly prioritizing our fertility, not our quality of life. But this only happens if they believe us at all: often, they shrug off our pain as normal or due to our "low pain tolerance." We as patients know the deep emotional and physical pain of having our symptoms dismissed.

Women, historically, have been dismissed and deemed hysterical by medical providers and those around them. In fact, the word hysteria comes from the word "hystera," the Greek word for uterus. In ancient Egypt, scholars thought that women suffered from hysteria because their uterus was out of place, wandering about the abdomen. The treatments all centered around trying to get the uterus back into place. In ancient Greece, physicians adapted this idea, and added that women with anxiety, fatigue, pain, heavy menstrual bleeding, and infertility were suffering because they were not married and having children, causing their uterus to wander.

How many of these women had endometriosis or other painful reproductive health issues?

In recent history, endometriosis was known as a working white women's disease, primarily impacting white women who delayed having children because of their career. This not only shamed working women, but also is racist in nature, completely excluding Black women and women of color from diagnosis.

One might think that these ridiculous, antiquated notions are squarely in the past. Except, these misinformed, patriarchal, patient-blaming beliefs clearly influence today's providers, especially those that are overly concerned about our fertility. After I had a traumatic C-section, my doctor told me I better hurry up and have another baby before the endometriosis spreads again. My doctor believed that I had a small window to try to get pregnant again and also that pregnancy would help all of the devastating symptoms I was having.

Endometriosis itself is still thought of by many providers as "the wandering womb," albeit with a more modern twist. Instead of the uterus itself escaping, it's the *lining* that has started roving throughout our bodies. When I questioned my OB/GYN regarding suitable hormone replacement therapy for endometriosis patients in perimenopause, she told me that since my uterus was gone, my endometriosis was also gone, as the lining of my uterus would not be spreading (wandering) anymore. I awkwardly had to explain that endometriosis by nature exists outside of the uterus, and a hysterectomy is not a cure.

When hormonal medications, repeated laparoscopic ablation surgeries, and finally a hysterectomy, do not cure our pain, fatigue, and other symptoms, we are at risk of being seen as hysterical, and our pain is now looked at as a mental health issue. These views can be extremely harmful to all women, but especially Black women and those who are a part of the LGBTQIA+ communities who are even more at risk of being dismissed, misdiagnosed and mistreated.

The worst part is, these providers are just following the antiquated, patriarchal standards of care that medical organizations outline, most often created without the input of endometriosis multidisciplinary specialists or patient advocates. The standards of care, written by organizations who deem themselves leaders in women's healthcare, often feel like they protect their own providers more than the patients they serve. Antiquated standards of care harm the reproductive health of the patients they serve, more than protect it.

Shame and Stigma

The shame and stigma associated with having challenges with physical intimacy or struggling to have a baby can deter us from speaking with our providers, family, and friends about the situation. In many cultures it is taboo to even talk about these things, truly making patients feel isolated. Opening up about painful sex is really hard. Sharing the pain of not being able to get pregnant or losing a pregnancy takes a lot of vulnerability and can feel risky as you hope the person hearing the information responds with empathy and validation.

These topics can make others uncomfortable and at times the responses from the most well-meaning loved ones leave us feeling worse. I once opened up to an older family member about my continued pregnancy losses after having my daughter. She responded, "Well, at least you have your daughter." At first, I felt shame and guilt for feeling devastated about my losses, until I remembered that I can feel grateful for my daughter while also feeling sad all at the same time. I realized my family members' response was coming from a place of discomfort in holding my feelings around this topic.

Certain cultures and religions put further pressure on women to sexually please their spouses and create babies, linking it to their purpose in life. Some people absurdly believe that women who do not have children hold a lesser value or opinion than those with children. The phrase, "Your body, my choice," has echoed throughout toxic corners of social media for some time now. These attitudes reflect a desire to control women and their bodies, as well as shame women who may not follow a certain lifestyle. These thoughts also pick at the emotional scars of women who may have struggled to have babies and ended their journey child-free. The boastful declaration that men control women's bodies is triggering for so many, including those who have suffered sexual violence, or who struggled to get a lifesaving abortion in their state. There is a deep lack of empathy for and cruelty towards women reflected in these attitudes and behaviors towards sexual and reproductive health.

As endometriosis advocates continue to fight for better standards of care from medical organizations like the American College of Obstetricians and Gynecologists (ACOG), we also feel deeply they are saying back to us, "Your body, our choice." This lack of listening and accountability from these medical organizations trickles down and impacts our care in the exam room. It took a longstanding social media campaign led by patients to highlight how painful IUD insertions could be to start a conversation about needed pain management. We routinely feel pain and discomfort during gynecological visits, treatments, and diagnostic tests. I have been on the exam table in only a sheet and a cropped smock, trying not to crawl out of my skin, with tears coming down my eyes, as the provider exclaimed in a frustrated tone, "This shouldn't hurt!" or, "You really have to relax!" These repeated invasive experiences that so many of us endure are humiliating and painful.

I understand that our pain may make providers uncomfortable, and they are frustrated that we aren't getting better. But are they more uncomfortable or frustrated than we are? Why isn't empathy their first reaction? How they react can reduce trauma or add to it.

To reduce shame and stigma surrounding sexuality and reproductive health, feminist perspectives teach that menstruation is natural and empowering. Menstrual product advertising executives capitalized on this, showing us being able to play soccer, jump, and laugh during that time of the month. Equality for women means that our bodies, and particularly our periods, do not make us less capable of doing things that men can. Sex is also presented as something empowering and pleasurable, with women being able to choose when and if to have a family through birth control and access to abortion. Fertility, pregnancy, childbirth and menopause are natural occurrences that should not hold us back or slow us down. There is the idea that women can have it all and do it all.

However, this narrative can alienate those of us who need extra time off or support for our painful periods, infertility treatments, miscarriages, or difficult births and postpartum. Due to the longstanding work of dedicated patient advocates, light is being shone on the challenges that some of us experience with our sexual and reproductive health. We as a society must embrace the idea that everyone is different and just because you may not have had any challenges in these areas, there are millions of others who do. Also, these challenges do not make us less capable or competent than others who struggle with medical conditions. Hopefully we continue to move towards a culture of empathy, when it comes to holding space for those experiencing sexual and reproductive health challenges. From providers within the exam rooms, to school policies and corporate benefits, and even religious ideologies, leading with empathy will improve reproductive health and reduce sexual and medical trauma.

Sexual Dysfunction

Honestly, I would rather not have sex and actually would rather avoid physical intimacy. Intercourse or any kind of penetration is painful. Having an orgasm is painful. The pain lasts long after intimacy is over. Nine out of ten times I also get a urinary tract infection after intercourse. Also, if I am feeling bloated, am super exhausted and having diarrhea, physical intimacy is the last thing on my mind. When I was dating my first boyfriend in high school, I often ignored my physical pain and lack of desire to be a "good girlfriend." He didn't understand why I never initiated sex and took it personally. We eventually broke up because of it. I just started learning about endometriosis from a friend of mine who just got diagnosed. I think I may have it too. It would explain a lot.
  –Lindsey, 19

Sexual Dysfunction Defined

The incredibly awkward sex talk that I received from my mom when I was a teenager was brief and centered around the palpable fear of getting pregnant. It was more of a talk than my own mother got from her mother, which was nonexistent. As women with combined decades of reproductive health challenges, I wish we both had been given the information and tools to understand that yes, there are inherent risks to consider when having sex, but also that sex should not be painful, but fun and pleasurable, that it is okay to advocate for your own sexual needs, and that if sex doesn't feel good emotionally or physically, it is okay to abstain and seek professional support. Had I been given this information, as well as an earlier endometriosis diagnosis, I know my first sexual experiences would have been dramatically different. When your first sexual experiences are painful, and continue to be over time, it leaves an imprint on the brain and the body that becomes harder and harder to rewire.

Sexual dysfunction occurs when there are persistent, recurrent challenges with sexual response, orgasm, or pain. These factors can be both emotional and physical in nature, as well as situational.

Mental health factors:

- stress
- depression
- anxiety
- shame
- guilt
- premenstrual syndrome, premenstrual dysphoric disorder
- past sexual or medical trauma.

Physical health factors:

- pregnancy
- perimenopause or menopause
- postpartum period
- substance use disorder
- other conditions, diseases, and medical treatments.

Endometriosis and Sexual Dysfunction

Over 50% of endometriosis patients will experience sexual dysfunction. As you can see, this doesn't affect everyone, but there is a high prevalence. For many of us, painful sex can be an important indicator of endometriosis. Endometriosis and its common comorbidities, such as adenomyosis and female bladder pain syndrome, can cause dyspareunia, or persistent or recurrent pain with vaginal insertion, penetration, thrusting, pain with orgasm as well as pain that can linger for hours after.

Endometriotic lesions cause pain, fibrosis and inflammation. When you have pain with vaginal insertion, penetration, thrusting, and pain with orgasm, these can be signs that these lesions and the surrounding inflamed tissue are being agitated. The most likely pain generators are lesions in the rectovaginal area, the cervix, the posterior and anterior cul-de-sacs, uterosacral ligaments as well as other areas. And when you have recurrent pain during physical intimacy, this can lead to stress and anxiety surrounding physical intimacy, which only increases pain.

Endometriosis in the pelvis, especially if left untreated for years, can cause pelvic floor dysfunction, which can also contribute to sexual dysfunction. Chronic pain can both weaken and tighten the pelvic floor, restricting its ability to contract and relax, causing a lot of tension.

Endometriosis can also cause hypersensitive trigger points in the pelvis. Pelvic pain caused by endometriosis affects the pelvic nerves, surrounding connective tissue, and musculoskeletal system. Even when surgeons remove the endometriosis, you can still have lingering pain due to continued pelvic muscle spasms, nerve pain and formed pain pathways that need to be reset.

Certain medications prescribed to minimize endometriosis symptoms, such as oral contraceptives, Depo-Provera, and Lupron can also impact sex drive and cause vaginal dryness as well. If you've had your ovaries removed (an oophorectomy) along with a hysterectomy, a change in hormones can also cause a decrease in sexual response or desire, as well as vaginal changes and dryness that can cause painful sex.

The Toll of Sexual Dysfunction

Sexual dysfunction is linked to stress, anxiety and depression in endometriosis patients. It can impact our self-esteem, and the desire or capacity to seek out romantic relationships or feel connected to our sexuality. A body filled with endometriosis is a body in pain and a body in crisis. When we are in pain and in crisis, it's difficult to muster up the physical and emotional capacity for sexual intimacy and desire. The challenge is that some of us suffer for decades without support or interventions for our endometriosis, having a huge impact on sexual health and worsening our mental health.

Sexual dysfunction can have a profound impact on even the most healthy relationships. While men have more medications (which insurance almost always covers) for sexual dysfunction, and providers have tried to reduce the stigma and normalize it, we have fewer options and are left to suffer in silence. Maybe you feel that even though sex is painful, you are unable to open up to your partner about it or refuse sexual interactions. There are some cultures and religions that frown upon or even forbid women to refuse sex from their husbands, exposing them to sexual coercion or intimate partner violence. If you're actively trying to have a baby and going through infertility, you might be feeling more pressure to suffer through sexual dysfunction as the dream to build a family feels at stake. The pain of having sex, the intrusiveness and pain of fertility treatments and the incredible stress of it all takes quite a physical and emotional toll and profoundly impacts sexual health.

Support for Endometriosis and Sexual Dysfunction

Removing endometriotic lesions and the surrounding fibrosis and scar tissue can help if you are struggling with painful sex. But, it is only one step in the healing process, as even with the disease gone, pain can still remain. An expert pelvic floor physical therapist will help strengthen your pelvic floor, increase mobility, release trigger points, and reduce tension, which can restore not only sexual function, but sexual confidence and improved relaxation as well.

Gynecological providers have the capability to help with sexual dysfunction and to also not make it worse. If you can find a provider that leads with empathy and curiosity when it comes to your observed pain, this will lead to earlier interventions and diagnosis. Look for a provider that implements trauma-informed care to make pelvic exams and invasive testing less painful and less traumatic, while offering appropriate pain relief before exams, diagnostic tests and procedures to reduce your emotional and physical trauma and sexual dysfunction. Your provider can also recommend pelvic floor therapy, and prescribe medications that can help with vaginal dryness or relaxing the pelvic floor.

Mental health support is also an important part of multidisciplinary care for sexual dysfunction. Cognitive behavioral therapy or EMDR are two therapeutic interventions that are great tools in helping with the fear and anxiety that can come from having a history of endometriosis or other reproductive health challenges, sexual trauma, medical trauma, or painful sex. Therapists can also help if you have anxiety, depression, and self-esteem issues related to sexual dysfunction. For those in a relationship, couples therapy with an experienced sex therapist can help support communication between couples who have had challenges in this area. Exploring other ways to be physically intimate, and strengthening emotional intimacy outside of intercourse is also important.

I cannot think of a pejorative word designated to men who refuse sex because they are uncomfortable. Women are more often subjected to shame or guilt for refusing sexual intimacy, even being labeled a "prude" or "tease." RAINN, the Rape, Abuse & Incest National Network reports that 1 out of every 6 American women has been the victim of an attempted or completed rape in her lifetime. It is crucial for those with endometriosis who have been a victim of sexual assault and abuse to have added support, consideration, and validation as they navigate their trauma as well as their physical pain. It is crucial for all patients, especially for endometriosis patients, for it to always be acceptable to refuse sex.

Supporting patients, believing their pain, offering them education and quality care, while holding those who harm them accountable, whether it be a sexual predator or an insensitive and misinformed provider, are the paths forward to improving sexual health and reducing sexual trauma which will also help restore sexual function.

Infertility

While all of the symptoms of endometriosis were incredibly difficult, the impact that endometriosis had on my reproductive health altered my life's path and made me feel broken in a way that took a long time to heal. I had always dreamed of becoming a mother. For years, I put my hurting body through fertility treatments. I was left emotionally, physically, and financially drained. Endometriosis stole my dream. Through grief, I had to reimagine my entire life.
  –Melissa, age 36

Infertility Defined

I can remember how fast and loud my heart was beating as I sat in the waiting room at my first reproductive endocrinologist appointment. I was terrified. Somehow, my anxiety convinced me that the doctor was going to give me the devastating news on the spot that I could never have children. I averted the glances of others in the waiting room, fearful that someone was going to recognize me, as we had told no one about our first appointment. Twenty minutes later, I had the most painful and humiliating pelvic exam I ever experienced, as my doctor entered my rectum and my cervix, with different fingers, at the same time, to try to assess my uterus. The years of painful, invasive and costly diagnostic tests and treatments, failures and successes, and losses that infertility brought me is something that is forever imprinted on my body, mind and soul.

The American Society for Reproductive Medicine defines infertility as a disease or condition characterized by the inability to achieve a successful pregnancy, which can be accompanied by the need for medical intervention to achieve a successful pregnancy. For those without any factors that indicate infertility or a need for medical intervention, they recommend that patients under 35 years of age should seek an evaluation after trying to conceive for a year, and those over the age of 35 years should seek an evaluation after trying to conceive for six months.

Endometriosis and Infertility

Not everyone with endometriosis suffers from infertility, but the American Society of Reproductive Medicine estimates that 30–50% of women with endometriosis suffer from infertility and 25–50% of women with infertility have endometriosis. There are multiple factors that can contribute to infertility in endometriosis patients.

- Endometriosis can cause pain with intercourse, making it emotionally and physically difficult to try to conceive.
- Endometriosis, and the fibrosis, scar tissue and adhesions it causes, can lead to anatomical disruptions to the reproductive process. Endometriosis can impact fallopian tubes disrupting ovulation and fertilization, also putting patients at risk for ectopic pregnancies.

- Endometriomas, endometriotic cysts on the ovaries, as well as ovarian adhesions, can impact ovulation, egg quality and quantity.
- Endometriosis anywhere in the pelvis causes oxidative stress and inflammation, releasing cytokines into the peritoneal fluid. This inflammation can impact egg quality, fertilization, and implantation.
- Comorbidities common to endometriosis patients such as adenomyosis, fibroids, or autoimmune diseases, like Hashimoto's disease, can also contribute to infertility.
- Unexplained fertility is an especially challenging diagnosis that can happen in up to 30% of couples trying to conceive. Because some endometriosis can be asymptomatic, or symptoms of endometriosis go unreported or missed by providers, endometriosis specialists have reported a prevalence of endometriosis after diagnostic laparoscopic confirmation of disease with those who had been diagnosed previously with unexplained infertility.
- For some endometriosis patients, the paths to family building include adoption, exploring donor eggs, donor embryos, or surrogacy due to the impact endometriosis has had on their fertility.
- Some patients with endometriosis make the deeply personal decision not to pursue family building due to the impact of their disease or decide to stop after attempts at family building did not work out.

The Toll of Infertility

Physically Intrusive and Painful

Struggling with infertility while also having endometriosis can be incredibly difficult on our bodies. With up to 50% of women with infertility diagnosed with endometriosis, it is disappointing how little the healthcare community and providers discuss the physical pain of the diagnostic tests and treatments. Depending on where the endometriosis is located, transvaginal ultrasounds, which are common during fertility treatments, can be painful. If your ovary is adhered to your pelvic wall, the stimulation process during IVF can be very painful. Diagnostic tests and procedures that involve speculum insertions or catheter insertions can be especially uncomfortable for endometriosis patients. Some endometriosis patients report feeling generally unwell on fertility medications, with symptoms flaring.

Emotionally Devastating

Endometriosis patients who also experience infertility are particularly vulnerable to anxiety and depression. If you dream of having a family, the fear and uncertainty that comes with not knowing if or how it will happen has a huge impact on your mental health. If you have a history of anxiety, this uncertainty can feel all-consuming. The pressure from family, friends, and society to have babies, and the intrusive ways it is a seemingly benign conversation starter, can make family events and social gatherings painful. If you come from a culture or religion where a woman's whole identity and purpose is to have babies, adapting to the infertility diagnosis can be especially challenging. The mental load of navigating and scheduling medical appointments is exhausting.

Endometriosis and infertility, and the physical pain and lack of control over our physical autonomy creates disconnect between our physical bodies, our identity and emotions. There is also an associated risk of postpartum depression and/or anxiety with those who undergo fertility treatments, although more research needs to be done to explore this association. No matter how your family building is resolved, grief is always a part of infertility.

Medical Racism and Homophobia Impacting Care

Black women are twice as likely to experience infertility than white women, yet are far less likely to receive treatment and be referred to treatment. Even when undergoing treatment, Black women are less likely to achieve pregnancy and have lower live birth rates. Also, patients report a lack of culturally competent care while in treatment. Due to experiencing racism, stigma, dismissal and mistreatment in the medical industrial complex, Black women are also less likely to seek out care.

Patients in the LGBTQIA+ community may face many obstacles when accessing infertility care. For some in the community, having to use a donor may include more planning and expenses. Patients are also at risk of discrimination by providers and may not feel welcomed at the clinic. More research needs to be done on endometriosis, infertility, and transgender men in order to provide them with competent and compassionate fertility care.

Financially Draining

Obtaining multidisciplinary care for endometriosis can be financially draining and trying to navigate infertility care can be incredibly overwhelming. Advocates in certain states have fought for and achieved state mandates for some level of fertility benefits to be covered, but access to care and coverage dramatically differ from employer to employer, and state to state. For many endometriosis patients, working enough hours to get healthcare coverage is a challenge in itself. For those who need to use donor eggs or embryos, a surrogate, or build a family through adoption, due to the impact of endometriosis on fertility and its comorbidities, the financial burden can be even higher, with coverage more elusive. Often, they feel like they have to make impossible choices when it comes to affording care, feeling like they do not have options to pursue treatments.

There are lists of companies that are known to be more financially supportive of fertility treatments and adoption in their benefit packages, with some offering remote work. There are also nonprofits dedicated to providing scholarships to patients who are struggling to afford their family building journey.

Access to Care

Just like when trying to find an endometriosis specialist, not every town or city has providers that offer fertility treatments. Personhood bills, which define personhood at the time of fertilization, have made patients and providers concerned about restricted access to IVF in some states. In 2024, Alabama granted embryos the same right to life as children, temporarily halting IVF procedures in the state. Later, an IVF immunity law was passed to afford some protections to IVF patients and providers, but the fear that family building options could be restricted remains. In 2024, a bill to protect access to IVF failed to pass again in the US Senate.

Support for Endometriosis and Infertility

Infertility and endometriosis have a profound impact on just about every aspect of life! Having support and an excellent multidisciplinary team is crucial to navigate both of these challenging and devastating medical conditions, along with any comorbidities.

Even at the most prestigious and well-attended endometriosis conferences, you may find differing opinions on how best to navigate endometriosis and infertility. As the patient going through it, the most important perspective is yours! Your priorities, your goals, your physical and emotional well-being should always be at the forefront, and your team is there to support you!

My OB/GYN was the first person that I reached out to regarding my infertility. My partner and I were having no luck getting pregnant on our own. I had a feeling that something was wrong. I had been experiencing pain with my periods for some time and was feeling generally unwell. I also had a family history of recurrent pregnancy loss. A supportive OB/GYN would have validated my pain, suspected endometriosis and referred me to both an endometriosis specialist and a reproductive endocrinologist in a timely manner.

My OB/GYN was unfortunately not very helpful. She dismissed my pain and told me, at the age of 26, that I was too young to be worried about infertility. I pressed for a referral to a reproductive endocrinologist.

A Reproductive Endocrinologist and Infertility Subspecialist (REI) is also known as a fertility specialist. They are OB/GYNs that have additional training in reproductive medicine, diagnosing and treating all the causes of infertility. If you are an endometriosis patient concerned about fertility, experienced infertility, or interested in preserving fertility, an REI can be an important member of your multidisciplinary team. An endometriosis-informed REI should be able to suspect endometriosis through an exam and a thorough patient history.

Through different diagnostic tests, REIs check:

- your baseline fertility
- your ovarian reserve and hormone levels
- the inside of your uterine cavity and fallopian tubes
- other comorbidities that can cause infertility, such as PCOS, genetic factors, thyroid issues.

REIs vs. Endo Excision Specialists

Before IVF was as accessible, REIs used surgery to remove and treat endometriosis to improve fertility. Some were even considered pioneers in the field of microsurgery and minimally invasive surgery. But, in recent years, improvement in IVF outcomes for endometriosis patients, poor surgery compensation, and more gynecologists focusing on minimally invasive gynecological surgical training have encouraged REIs to focus more on assisted reproductive technology than endometriosis surgery. They believe that they can work around the impact endometriosis has on fertility through fertility treatments, and then being pregnant is the best thing to calm the disease.

An endometriosis excision specialist believes that excising all of the disease they can see, restoring anatomy, and reducing inflammation in the pelvis, will not only improve fertility, but also improve quality of life and organ function. Unlike the majority of REIs, an endometriosis excision specialist excises disease impacting the reproductive organs, preserving fertility, and spends time and attention on all impacted organs. Some studies have shown that surgically removing endometriosis can improve spontaneous pregnancy rates and improve rates of success with IVF. Ideally, an endometriosis excision specialist and an REI will work together with you, providing informed consent on all treatment options, helping you decide what course of treatment best aligns with your goals and your physical, emotional, and financial well-being. Some patients will need to utilize fertility treatments even after excision.

Multidisciplinary care such as pelvic floor physical therapy, acupuncture, and functional medicine with practitioners who have an understanding of endometriosis and infertility can also be great additions to your team. Mental health support is crucial as well. Both infertility and endometriosis can cause anxiety, depression, and are incredibly stressful. Both endometriosis and infertility can be isolating, so peer support groups can be an important source of support during this time as well because it can be hard to open up to family and friends who don't have an understanding of what you are going through. For the BIPOC and LGBTQIA+ communities, finding peer support is especially important as you navigate unique challenges to family building.

Pregnancy Loss

We were so happy to get the positive pregnancy test. We had been casually trying to get pregnant for a while with no luck. My periods would come and not only would they be heavy and physically excruciating, they were a painful emotional reminder that we were not pregnant. So many of my friends were pregnant or had new babies and I didn't know why that wasn't happening for us. When we finally got a positive test, all of the anxiety and stress melted away as we shared the news with close family and friends. I already felt so much love towards and had so many dreams for this tiny being that was smaller than a blueberry. When I started bleeding heavily a week later I was in shock. At what was supposed to be our appointment to see the heartbeat, my doctor confirmed I was having a miscarriage. I have never felt so sad and alone.
–Ciara, 26

Pregnancy Loss Defined

For a span of years in my thirties, I felt like my sick body was a hospice for genetically challenged embryos. I endured miscarriage after miscarriage, often after transferring what we thought were healthy embryos that held so much promise. My struggling body, pumped up with fertility medications while filled with endometriosis and adenomyosis, painfully labored through each loss. The despair, shame, guilt, and physical and emotional anguish I felt with each loss was all-consuming.

Pregnancy loss can be a physically and emotionally devastating experience that happens in at least 1 in 4 pregnancies. Although it is prevalent, it can be incredibly difficult to talk openly about it, leaving those who go through it to often suffer in silence. There are a few different types of losses that patients can experience, each difficult and painful in their own ways.

- A pregnancy loss, also known as a miscarriage or spontaneous abortion, is a nonviable intrauterine pregnancy up to 20 weeks' gestation.
- An ectopic pregnancy is when the fertilized egg develops outside of the uterus, usually in the fallopian tubes. This is potentially life-threatening.
- A biochemical pregnancy is when pregnancy hormones are detected, but the embryo stops developing within the first five weeks of pregnancy, before the fetus can be seen on an ultrasound.
- An early pregnancy loss is a miscarriage before 13 weeks of pregnancy, as defined by the ACOG.
- A recurrent miscarriage is diagnosed when two or more early miscarriages occur.
- A second trimester loss or a late miscarriage is a loss after 13 weeks and before 24 weeks' gestation.
- A stillbirth is when a baby or fetus dies at or after 20 or 28 weeks of pregnancy in the uterus or during birth.

Endometriosis and Pregnancy Loss

While not all endometriosis patients will experience pregnancy loss, endometriosis patients are associated with a greater risk for pregnancy loss and recurrent pregnancy loss because of the structural issues, inflammation, and immunological factors associated with the disease.

- Endometriosis patients are at a greater risk for developing ectopic pregnancies. Disease and adhesions can impact the fallopian tubes, preventing the fertilized egg from implanting in

the uterus. As the pregnancy grows, the fallopian tube can rupture, which can lead to internal bleeding that requires urgent surgery or risks death.
- Inflammation may impact the endometrium, the egg and embryo quality, as well as the placenta development, leading to a greater risk of pregnancy loss.
- Immunological and genetic factors may contribute to a higher likelihood of pregnancy loss, including euploid loss in those with endometriosis.
- Adenomyosis, fibroids, and uterine anomalies such as bicornuate uterus, are associated comorbidities with endometriosis that impact the uterus, which are also associated with a greater rate of miscarriage.
- Black women have nearly a twofold increased risk of miscarriage as compared to white women. Widespread racial disparities, including delays in getting care due to medical racism, are factors that may contribute to this increase.

We don't have enough research or a general understanding among providers and society alike about the physical and emotional pain that comes with endometriosis and pregnancy loss. For those of us who have endometriosis and have experienced pregnancy loss, we truly understand how painful and devastating it can be.

Thanks to the tireless work of advocates over the years, the physical pain associated with endometriosis is starting to be widely accepted and understood. While endometriosis isn't just killer cramps, severe pain with periods can be a hallmark symptom. Miscarriages for those without endometriosis are associated with heavier cramping, clotting and bleeding that can last longer than a period. It's not hard then to make a leap and say that miscarriages are most likely even more physically excruciating for those with endometriosis and uterine comorbidities, like adenomyosis.

To reduce physical discomfort and trauma, professional gynecological associations and providers must work together with patient advocates to develop a standard pain management protocol for anyone experiencing a miscarriage, but especially for those of us that are prone to pain, heavy bleeding and clotting with menstruation due to disease.

The Toll of Pregnancy Loss

No matter when your pregnancy loss happens, it is deeply distressing. In fact, 1 in 3 patients develop post-traumatic stress disorder. Those of us who experience pregnancy loss may experience anxiety or depression and feelings of overwhelming grief. This grief often happens in isolation, as those around us may not know about the loss or know how to be supportive. Platitudes from well-meaning friends and family such as, "It just wasn't meant to be," "Everything happens for a reason," or, "At least you know you can get pregnant," (all of which I have personally been told!) may further upset you, if you are looking for a safe space to process emotions. Pregnancy loss after fertility treatments can add additional emotional and physical pain and emotional distress.

The Supreme Court's *Dobbs v. Jackson Women's Health Organization* decision in June 2022, which marked the removal of the constitutional right to abortion in the US, has complicated access to miscarriage care in certain states. Patients who need or desire intervention or management during their miscarriage, either for life threatening infection or bleeding, unexpected complications, or just to reduce mental or physical trauma by helping the body process the loss, may face obstacles due to the legal limitations placed upon providers by state politicians. These restrictions have tragically not only added to the emotional trauma of people experiencing loss, but in some cases, a delay in needed emergency miscarriage care, resulted in not only a loss of fertility, but a loss of life.

Support for Endometriosis and Pregnancy Loss

If you're experiencing pregnancy loss, you can ask your gynecologist for a referral to a reproductive endocrinologist or a reproductive immunologist to get more information and see if there is any further support your body needs to achieve a healthy pregnancy.

A reproductive endocrinologist can provide more information and support for pregnancy loss. They can test for:

- thyroid issues
- chromosomal abnormalities
- genetic factors
- hormonal factors such as low progesterone
- autoimmune conditions
- fibroids
- uterine anomalies
- adenomyosis
- scarred fallopian tubes.

An endometriosis excision specialist excises disease and reduces inflammation in the pelvis, which may be contributing to pregnancy loss. A skilled surgeon will remove fibroids and potentially treat an adenoma of the uterus or a uterine anomaly during surgery. Also, during surgery, they can assess and remove scarred fallopian tubes to reduce the risk of an ectopic pregnancy.

If you struggle with recurrent pregnancy loss, a reproductive immunologist is a great addition to your multidisciplinary team. Reproductive immunologists look at how the immune system interacts with the reproductive system, and they can see if any inflammation caused by your endometriosis is affecting your pregnancy outcomes or IVF results. Because endometriosis has a greater association with certain autoimmune diseases, one or more of these may be unknowingly impacting your pregnancy outcomes; a reproductive immunologist can investigate these causes as well.

Maternal fetal medicine specialists are trained to help patients who are at risk for, or have been identified as having, a high-risk pregnancy. If you have a history of recurrent pregnancy loss, are of advanced maternal age (35 or older), or have a chronic, preexisting health condition like diabetes, inflammatory bowel disease, autoimmune disease, or kidney disease, you might be referred to a maternal fetal medicine specialist. While some endometriosis patients do not experience pregnancy loss or pregnancy complications, due to the increased risk, you may still benefit from their insights.

Multidisciplinary care can be incredibly helpful if you're going through pregnancy loss. Pelvic floor physical therapy, acupuncture, and functional medicine are tools that can help support your body as it heals from pregnancy loss.

Having support for any grief, anxiety, depression, or PTSD that can arise after a pregnancy loss is crucial. Pregnancy loss is not your fault, although it is hard not to internalize blame. You can seek out a mental health provider familiar with pregnancy loss or one of many virtual and in-person support groups. Connecting with others who have gone through this can help you feel less alone and experience shared grief. Through individual and group support, you can learn to process your grief and explore personal rituals to mark the loss of the pregnancy, as well as mourn anniversaries as time passes. Providers who are trauma-informed will best support you through this sensitive and vulnerable time.

Pregnancy Complications

> I should have known my body was going to fail us. My body has been failing me since I got my period in the fifth grade. Years of bleeding and pain, followed by years of fertility treatments to finally get pregnant only to have my body fail us. At 28 weeks I started having contractions. Because of dealing with the pain of endometriosis for so many years, I almost didn't even notice the contractions. My doctors and I tried everything to stop what felt inevitable. My little preemie is doing okay in the NICU. I know that I am very lucky that she has made it this far, but it is still hard. I can't help but feel like my body failed her.
> —Meg, 40

Like many of us, I was told that if I just got pregnant, my endometriosis would be in remission and it would be smooth sailing from there! Also like many of us, that was definitely not my experience! A lot of my pregnancy was filled with pelvic pain as my body adjusted to the growing baby. I experienced spotting and for six weeks I could only eat rice, bananas and applesauce because of severe gastrointestinal issues. At my 34-week appointment, my ultrasound showed that I was having Braxton Hicks contractions and my baby was breached. My doctor told me it was nothing to worry about. My daughter was born 24 hours later through an emergency cesarean section.

The more I talk to other patients, the more I hear about their similar pregnancy and birth stories. The more I learn about endometriosis, the more I understand the pregnancy complications associated with endometriosis and wonder why no provider had ever warned me of the potential of developing these issues.

Pregnancy Complications Defined

A pregnancy can be classified as complicated for a multitude of reasons and it indicates that you and the fetus are at risk and need to be more closely monitored. A multiple gestation pregnancy, such as twins or triplets, can be considered a complicated pregnancy or if the pregnant person has any health issues, ranging from mental health challenges such as depression to chronic health conditions such as diabetes. Also, if there are health issues with the fetus, a pregnancy can be considered at risk.

Maternal-fetal medicine specialists are OB/GYNs who have additional training to support you through high-risk pregnancies and complications. If you have a preexisting chronic health condition such as high blood pressure, heart disease, thyroid disease, or depression, or if you are at risk for preterm labor, you will most likely be referred to a maternal-fetal medicine specialist by your OB/GYN or midwife. If you develop a new, not preexisting condition, during pregnancy, such as preeclampsia or placenta previa, your OB/GYN or midwife may also refer you to a maternal-fetal medicine specialist.

Endometriosis and Pregnancy Complications

Just like not all endometriosis patients are going to experience infertility or pregnancy loss, not all patients are going to experience pregnancy complications. Actually, the story that many patients are told by providers is that pregnancy helps the symptoms of endometriosis, and "gives your body a break." But there is *no* strong research to support this. Hormonal changes in pregnancy may help some, but also may exacerbate symptoms for others. One has to wonder if this theory comes from that ancient belief that if there is a baby in the womb it isn't wandering, causing pain and hysteria.

The research does show endometriosis patients undergo more pregnancy complications. Endometriosis patients have a higher incidence of:

- preterm labor and birth
- preeclampsia
- placenta previa
- placental abruption.

Currently, endometriosis patients who get pregnant spontaneously, or who graduate from the reproductive endocrinologist's office, are placed with a regular obstetric provider and not referred to a maternal-fetal medicine specialist. It could be beneficial to improve the standard of care for pregnant endometriosis patients, considering the potential risk factors associated with endometriosis and pregnancy.

Pain with pregnancy: For some endometriosis patients, pregnancy can be painful, especially in the first few months. If you think about the painful endometriotic lesions and scar tissue embedded throughout the pelvis, sticking organs together through adhesions, it's not hard to imagine that an ever growing uterus, putting pressure on and stretching and pulling all of these things, can cause pain.

Preterm labor and birth: A Danish study found that those with diagnosed endometriosis were more at risk for having preterm labor, as compared to those without endometriosis. Infertility treatments, fibroids, and adenomyosis also are associated with preterm labor. More research needs to be done to further understand these connections.

Uterine anomalies: There is an association between septate uteri, bicornuate uteri and endometriosis, with a higher incidence of those with endometriosis having these anomalies. Uterine anomalies can increase the risk of preterm labor, and for a baby being breech, increasing the chance of having a cesarean section.

Preeclampsia: Preeclampsia is characterized by high blood pressure and high levels of protein in the urine that can develop during pregnancy, usually after the 20th week of gestation. Research has shown an association between patients with endometriosis and a higher incidence of preeclampsia. Untreated, preeclampsia can be harmful to both the pregnant person and the baby, which can lead to an unplanned preterm birth.

Placenta previa: Research has shown a strong association between patients with endometriosis and a higher incidence of placenta previa. Placenta previa is when the placenta attaches to the uterus close to or over the cervix. Uterine anomalies or previous uterine surgeries are associated with placenta previa. Placenta previa causes vaginal bleeding usually after 20 weeks of gestation. Modified activities and careful monitoring will most likely be prescribed. Patients with placenta previa are more at risk of having preterm birth as well as a cesarean section.

Placental abruption: This is when the placenta separates from the inner wall of the uterus before birth. This separation can cause bleeding and pain in the pregnant person and can deprive the baby of oxygen and nutrients. The outcomes of placental abruption depend on how quickly the pregnant person can get intervention, how separate the placenta is, and how far along the pregnancy is. Medications to help develop the baby's brain and lungs, as well as monitored bed rest are interventions often used to support the pregnant person and baby. Patients with placenta abruption are more at risk of having preterm birth as well as a cesarean section.

Black birthing people are three times more likely to die from pregnancy complications than their white counterparts. They are also more likely to develop preeclampsia, have a higher rate of cesarean deliveries, as well as experience preterm birth than white birthing people. We know having endometriosis only increases these risk factors.

The Toll of Pregnancy Complications

If you suffered from pregnancy complications, you are more at risk for anxiety, depression, PTSD and medical trauma, and if you suffer perinatal complications you are more at risk of postpartum depression. Parents who experience preterm labor may have to have their babies stay in the NICU making them more prone to experience anxiety, stress, relationship strain, family stress, as well as financial strain. Giving birth to a preemie can increase risk of postpartum depression by 40% as compared to full-term babies. Recovering from complications such as an emergency cesarean section or preeclampsia takes time and can be challenging, with the recovering parent needing to take extra care as healing continues.

Support for Pregnancy Complications

If you experience pregnancy complications, your team can include a reproductive endocrinologist, an OB/GYN or midwife, and a maternal-fetal medicine specialist. You need a trauma-informed, compassionate, expert team to get you through your pregnancy as well as through postpartum healing. As an endometriosis patient, healing from pregnancy complications and a traumatic birth can take longer, as your body may already be struggling due to untreated disease.

You may also benefit from pelvic floor physical therapy, which can help your body heal from pregnancy complications.

Trying to heal from a traumatic birth, while also dealing with endometriosis, while also trying to take care of a newborn may feel incredibly overwhelming at times. Mental health support is crucial to help you process your grief and trauma and assess and treat postpartum depression or anxiety. Peer support groups can also help you feel less alone and help you process your experiences. The support of family and friends can also help you feel less isolated as well as help you with physical tasks as your body heals.

Perimenopause and Menopause

If there is one thing that providers know less about than endometriosis, it is perimenopause and menopause! It feels like a stressful repeat of the long road to my endometriosis diagnosis. I have all these symptoms that keep getting dismissed. I just keep getting told to exercise and eat better! None of my doctors seem to agree on what treatments to give me, or if I am even in perimenopause. I am having to

follow expert providers on social media and do all of my own research which is exhausting. If men experienced menopause I have to believe that there would be more research, more interventions, and a better standard of care!
—Anna, age 45

Perimenopause and Menopause Defined

Menopause is characterized by a decline in reproductive hormones, including estrogen, leading to a decline in fertility. Menopause starts the day after a full 12 months of no periods. From then on, you're considered "in menopause," "menopausal" or "postmenopausal." If you were born with ovaries, you will experience menopause, most likely between the ages of 45 and 55.

Perimenopause occurs during the years leading up to menopause and lasts anywhere from two to ten years. During perimenopause, reproductive hormones can fluctuate significantly. Black women and Latinas are reported to experience perimenopause earlier, for a longer period of time, and also with more intense symptoms.

Like endometriosis, the symptoms of perimenopause and menopause impact all parts of the body. Symptoms can include:

- hot flashes
- night sweats
- changes in sexual desire
- vaginal dryness
- headaches
- trouble sleeping
- trouble with concentration or memory
- dry skin and eyes
- changes in vision
- bone loss and osteoporosis
- challenges with dental health.

A decline in reproductive hormones also can lower serotonin levels, causing anxiety, depression, irritability, and mood swings. Elevated blood sugar and cholesterol can also impact a patient's health during this time.

Endometriosis, Perimenopause and Menopause

Similarly to endometriosis, the majority of providers do not get a robust education in perimenopause and menopause. There also is very little research in these areas. The research on endometriosis *and* menopause is even more scarce. Because of this, there has historically been much confusion surrounding endometriosis and menopause, leading patients to suffer needlessly. If you are like me, and had a hysterectomy, but kept one ovary to avoid surgical menopause, providers can be even more confused as to where you are on the perimenopause/menopause spectrum and how to best support you.

So much of the research surrounding endometriosis and treatments for the disease are based on stopping menstruation, or dramatically reducing estrogen levels inducing menopause-like symptoms, or surgically removing our ovaries and/or uterus to treat the disease. We are told time and again that if we can make it to menopause we will feel better. Some of us are even encouraged to go through surgically induced menopause to be able to find relief from all of our endometriosis symptoms.

Some people do feel better once they are in menopause. I often wonder how many of these people also had adenomyosis or other uterine-based conditions that did get better after menstruation stopped. We know that endometriosis, adhesions, fibrosis and inflammation exist in menopausal patients. Endometriosis excision specialists are operating more and more on highly symptomatic menopausal patients, finding significant disease; they even find disease in patients who have long had their uterus and even ovaries removed.

We need more research on how to support endometriosis patients in perimenopause and menopause. Providers are often conflicted on how to prescribe endometriosis patients hormone replacement therapy (HRT). For a long time, they thought giving endometriosis patients estrogen was too risky, as it may cause endometriosis recurrence. On top of that, the medical community thought in general that HRT was dangerous for the majority of people.

However, research shows that HRT has many benefits and for the majority of people, carries low risks. HRT can actually reduce perimenopause and menopause symptoms, as well as decrease bone loss and risk of cardiovascular disease.

Recent research also shows that HRT can benefit endometriosis patients. All patients, but especially younger patients who are going through primary ovarian insufficiency or surgically induced menopause, due to bilateral oophorectomy, can reduce their risk of developing osteoporosis, cardiovascular disease, cognitive decline, and dementia by taking HRT.

HRT has benefited me greatly, and I have had no uptick in my endometriosis symptoms as I had feared. But, I do wonder if the extensive endometriosis excision surgeries I had gotten to remove the majority of my disease has helped in that regard. More research needs to be done on endometriosis patients and menopause.

The Toll of Perimenopause and Menopause

For many of us that have endured endometriosis for years, going through perimenopause and menopause can be challenging. After years of feeling not in control of our bodies, perimenopause and menopause can feel like an extension of those feelings. Perimenopause can change periods in unpredictable ways, leading to frustration. Weight gain that seems difficult to lose, especially around the abdomen, can also feel incredibly frustrating and leaves us open to criticism by uneducated providers. If you've had extensive endometriosis excision and successful treatment and haven't felt endometriosis symptoms for years, urinary issues, including seeming recurrent urinary tract infections, bladder dysfunction, or lack of sexual desire or pain with intercourse may bring up confusion and anxiety surrounding symptoms. Are symptoms related to endometriosis or perimenopause?

The gaslighting, the lack of information and misinformation from providers can be very triggering to many of us who have already been through this with endometriosis.

If you have had your reproductive organs removed, you will go through perimenopause or menopause sooner and could have a tougher time emotionally adapting to these changes, especially if you were not emotionally prepared for the loss. You may be feeling sad that your fertility window has closed, especially if you were still processing your struggles to build a family. Or you may be feeling empowered and relieved to close your tumultuous chapter on fertility and menstruation.

Many times, providers who are not experts in care are the quickest to tell you to remove your uterus and ovaries. Often, so much endometriosis is left after these castrative surgeries. In these cases, you not only still have disease throughout your pelvis, but are then thrown into surgical menopause. It is devastating. Unfortunately, your provider will also most likely deny you hormone replacement therapy because they're afraid to "feed the endometriosis." The consequences of not referring you to an endometriosis excision expert who can remove more disease and may preserve your reproductive organs, or at least to providers who have a better handle on hormone replacement therapy, are catastrophic. These decisions, which are supported by outdated practice guidelines and ideas, have long-term consequences that not only impact your quality of life, but ultimately your lifespan, as risk of heart disease and bone loss increase.

One study found that those with endometriosis may have a 20% greater risk of heart attack and ischemic stroke than those without. Other research has linked coronary heart disease and hysterectomies, and further research has showed hysterectomies in younger patients before natural menopause is connected to cardiovascular disease. More research needs to be done around these associations. Endometriosis has serious, potential, long-term, life-threatening considerations. Providers and patients need to be aware of these potential risks and implement preventative measures.

Support for Perimenopause and Menopause

The Menopause Society has a lot of great resources for patients and providers alike. On their website, you can find a directory where patients can look up providers in their area who are certified in menopause through their organization. Research has shown that for the majority of patients, hormone replacement therapy can have many benefits, and endometriosis patients are not excluded from that.

There are also many providers on social media, who have also written books, that are speaking up about menopause. On social media and in endometriosis support groups, there are advocates speaking up about endometriosis and menopause, sharing what they have learned through trial and error. Talking to peers who are also going through perimenopause and menopause can help patients feel validated. It is also a way to share information to get optimal care. Just like with endometriosis care, becoming our own educated advocate and leaving providers who are dismissive, and finding ones that are supportive, are the best ways to get the support we need during this transformative time.

4

It's Almost Never Just Endo
Common Comorbidities

If It's Not One Thing, It's Another

It took me a long time to accept the possibility that endometriosis was causing my suffering. I finally gathered the courage—and resources—to have my extensive endometriosis excision surgery. I had hoped that it would be the key to getting my life back.

During surgery, my endometriosis specialist noticed that my uterus appeared to be soft and enlarged. She suspected I have adenomyosis. I was not ready to have a hysterectomy and before surgery had told her to preserve my uterus.

Months have passed since my surgery and while I am feeling better in some ways, I still am not feeling great. I spend so much time and resources going to different providers to support my body, but I feel like it only helps so much.

My periods are still very heavy and painful. I also recently had my thyroid checked and had to start medication for Hashimoto's disease, now my third diagnosed chronic health condition this year. While I am grateful that I have answers, I feel really discouraged. When will I feel better? Is this what the rest of my life will look like?

–Sam, age 28

Unfortunately, if you have endometriosis, you may be at a higher risk of experiencing other chronic health issues in your lifetime. While we need more research on the "why" this happens, we as patients know it is happening, as many of us are living that reality.

There are endometriosis patients that come to see me for mental health support who present with symptoms of hypermobile Ehlers-Danlos Syndrome. It is not unusual for patients to come in with unexplained infertility and pregnancy loss who are presenting with classic endometriosis symptoms. Post-endometriosis excision patients who have continued bladder pain may end up with a female bladder pain syndrome diagnosis after seeing a urologist. Just as with endometriosis, the road to diagnosis and treatment for these comorbidities can also be long, exhausting, time-consuming and expensive.

I too have struggled with multiple chronic health conditions throughout my life, including endometriosis, adenomyosis, fibroids, infertility, Hashimoto's disease, recurrent pregnancy loss, and migraines. During my last endocrinologist visit, my thyroid ultrasound showed visible scarring due to my Hashimoto's disease. My doctor asked me if I had been feeling more tired lately. I didn't know how to answer that. More tired than when I had pervasive endometriosis while going through years of fertility treatments and pregnancy loss? More tired than before my first endometriosis excision surgery? More tired than before I had my hysterectomy for my fibroids and adenomyosis? With much of that behind me, I feel better than I have in years. Yet, I am probably still more tired than your average person without chronic health issues. As patients with ongoing health issues, it is hard for us to know what healthy feels like.

There are certain chronic conditions that are considered more common among endometriosis patients. For patients and providers alike, it can be hard to pinpoint which illness is causing specific symptoms, leading to challenges in diagnosis and treatment.

Adenomyosis

I can remember lying on my bed, feeling weak, pale and in excruciating pain. It was like my uterus was trying to repeatedly and violently vomit up my period through my vagina. Every month, the week before my period, crippling anxiety would come, as I questioned how I would survive the impending bleeding and pain. I already had endured five pelvic surgeries by the time I was considering my hysterectomy for suspected adenomyosis and fibroids. After years of unsuccessful fertility treatments and pregnancy losses, I was ready to leave my family building journey behind. The amount of pain and bleeding I was experiencing throughout my cycle was breathtaking, often leaving me to wonder if I should head to the emergency room. Yet, the thought of enduring another surgery to remove my uterus was incredibly overwhelming.
–Veronica, age 36

Adenomyosis Defined

Adenomyosis is a disease that impacts the uterus. If you have adenomyosis, the tissue (endometrial glands and stroma) from the lining of your uterus starts to infiltrate the muscular portion of the wall of the uterus. Adenomyosis can be diffused throughout the uterus, with disease being scattered in multiple areas. Adenomyosis can also be focal, with the disease being concentrated in one spot. An adenomyoma is a well-defined lesion surrounded by normal myometrium. The abnormal presence of endometrial glands within the myometrium creates pain and inflammation, while impacting the uterus' ability to control menstrual bleeding.

Symptoms associated with adenomyosis:

- heavy bleeding and clotting during periods
- prolonged periods
- increased risk of anemia
- painful periods
- painful intercourse/penetration
- chronic pelvic pain
- bloating
- back pain
- leg pain
- fatigue
- increased risk of infertility
- increased risk of pregnancy loss
- increased risk of adverse birth outcomes/complications.

Symptoms that can overlap with endometriosis:

- painful periods
- painful intercourse/penetration
- chronic pelvic pain
- bloating
- back pain
- leg pain
- fatigue
- increased risk of infertility
- increased risk of pregnancy loss
- increased risk of adverse birth outcomes/complications.

Challenges to Diagnosing and Treating Adenomyosis

While adenomyosis is often thought of as a disease impacting those who are later in their childbearing years, it absolutely can impact adolescents, causing heavy pain and bleeding that is disruptive to their quality of life. The majority of the symptoms of adenomyosis tend to disappear with menopause, but there have been some reported cases of adenomyosis impacting postmenopausal patients.

You can suspect you have adenomyosis by assessing your symptoms. However, a pelvic MRI can be an effective imaging tool to diagnose adenomyosis, although this depends on the skills of the providers reading the images and how progressed the disease is. Just like with endometriosis, normal imaging does not always rule out the presence of adenomyosis.

Unfortunately for now, the only definitive cure for diffuse adenomyosis is a hysterectomy. For those who have an adenomyoma or focal adenomyosis, an extremely skilled surgeon may be able to remove the disease from the myometrium, although there can be subsequent pregnancy risks associated with that procedure.

A presacral neurectomy is a procedure that may relieve the pain from adenomyosis while preserving fertility. This is best performed by a highly skilled and experienced laparoscopic gynecological surgeon. The surgeon will cut the nerves coming from the uterus to disrupt the pain signals coming from the brain. A presacral neurectomy comes with many risks and is best done by a provider who routinely performs this procedure. Also, the benefits of the presacral neurectomy can be limited, as the pain can return in time.

Medical management, such as anti-inflammatory medications, combined hormonal contraceptives or progesterone-based intrauterine devices (IUDs) can be helpful tools to minimize pain and bleeding.

Uterine Fibroids

As a young Black woman, I kept being told that my pain is normal and something I needed to endure. I started gaining weight and was so badly bloated that I looked pregnant. I felt so tired all of the time.

I went through so many years of suffering without answers. I finally saw a specialist who was able to diagnose and treat my fibroids and endometriosis. I finally have relief, yet, I am upset that it took so long to get the care I needed.
 —Jasmine, age 26

Uterine Fibroids Defined

Uterine fibroids, also referred to as uterine myomas, are noncancerous tumors that form in and around the uterus. Intramural fibroids grow within the muscular wall of the uterus. Submucosal fibroids bulge into the uterine cavity. Subserosal fibroids form on the outside of the uterus. Uterine fibroids can be very small or grow as large as the size of a grapefruit, sometimes even bigger. Some people who have fibroids may be asymptomatic, but symptoms can be based on size, number, or location of the fibroids. Black women are more at risk for developing fibroids. If a close family member has fibroids, you may be more at risk for having them as well.

Symptoms associated with uterine fibroids:

- heavy bleeding and clotting during periods
- prolonged periods
- increased risk of anemia
- more frequent periods
- painful periods
- painful intercourse/penetration
- chronic pelvic pain
- bloating
- back pain
- fatigue
- increased risk of infertility
- increased risk of pregnancy loss
- increased risk of adverse birth outcomes/complications
- frequent urination or trouble urinating
- constipation.

Symptoms that can overlap with endometriosis:

- painful periods
- painful intercourse/penetration

- chronic pelvic pain
- bloating
- back pain
- fatigue
- increased risk of infertility
- increased risk of pregnancy loss
- increased risk of adverse birth outcomes/complications
- frequent urination or trouble urinating
- constipation.

Challenges to Diagnosing and Treating Uterine Fibroids

While Black women are more at risk for having uterine fibroids, fibroids can impact patients of *all* races. Due to the correlation between Black women and uterine fibroids, Black women are more at risk for having a delayed endometriosis and/or adenomyosis diagnosis, as providers can mistakenly attribute symptoms solely to fibroids. While fibroids are often thought of as impacting patients who are of reproductive age, they also impact adolescents. Some research suggests that those in perimenopause are most at risk for developing fibroids. Fibroids may shrink during menopause, although in some cases may still be problematic for patients.

Like with adenomyosis, you can suspect you have uterine fibroids based on your symptoms. For confirmation that you have fibroids, you'll need a vaginal or abdominal ultrasound. A pelvic MRI can definitively diagnose the size and location of any existing fibroids while a hysterosonography and hysterosalpingography can investigate the inside of the uterus and can diagnose any submucosal fibroids.

A hysterectomy has been a long recommended treatment for fibroids. Black women experience a higher rate of hysterectomies for benign conditions, and also experience a higher rate of hysterectomy complications. It is crucial to note there are more options for treatment and true informed consent includes being presented with all available options to help you with decision making.

A myomectomy is a fertility-sparing surgical procedure that removes the fibroid while keeping the uterus. A laparoscopic myomectomy may result in fewer adhesions than abdominal myomectomy (laparotomy). When undergoing this option, discuss with your provider if a power morcellator will be used to help remove it. Morcellation includes cutting the fibroid into smaller pieces before removal. If the fibroid is cancerous, morcellation could spread the cancer cells further.

The ACESSA procedure, also known as radiofrequency ablation, is a laparoscopic procedure in which the surgeon uses intense heat to burn the fibroids, destroying the tissue and improving symptoms. This procedure is not recommended if you are planning for future pregnancies or if you are at risk for cancer or malignancy.

Uterine artery embolization/uterine fibroid embolization is a non-surgical procedure in which the provider first maps out the fibroids and identifies the arteries supplying blood to them. Using a tiny catheter, they inject microparticles into those small arteries to block the flow of blood to the fibroid, which will cause it to shrink and die. Benefits and risks to your fertility and pregnancy vary depending on your individual situation, so it's best to discuss with your provider.

The sonata system is an ultrasound treatment for fibroids that does not involve any incisions. The device is inserted by the doctor through the vagina and into the uterus. It delivers radiofrequency energy to the fibroid, causing it to shrink over time and relieve symptoms. Like with embolization, you should discuss the benefits and risks to fertility and pregnancy with your provider.

Medical management, such as anti-inflammatory medications, combined hormonal contraceptives or progesterone-based intrauterine devices (IUDs) can be helpful tools to minimize pain and bleeding.

Interstitial Cystitis (IC)/Female Bladder Pain Syndrome (FBPS)

My friends always joke about me having to pee all of the time. I always have to know where the bathrooms are when we go out, and I tend to avoid places and situations where I know I won't be able to access a bathroom. I know it seems funny to them, but it is stressful struggling with endometriosis and female bladder pain syndrome. Endometriosis

excision of my bladder and ureters during surgery helped me in some ways, but I still get pain flares, particularly from my FBPS. I constantly have to watch what I eat and drink. Sometimes it feels like I have a chronic urinary tract infection. I often feel depressed. It's hard to be young and feel like my life is centered around managing these chronic conditions.
—Laura, age 22

Female Bladder Pain Syndrome Defined

Female bladder pain syndrome, previously referred to as interstitial cystitis, is a chronic, painful, inflammatory condition impacting the bladder that can lead to scarring or stiffening of the bladder and the reduced ability to hold urine. Why certain patients get FBPS is still largely unknown. Researchers have found there may be different types of FBPS:

1. A non-ulcerative form with pinpoint hemorrhages on the bladder wall.
2. An ulcerative form which includes red, bleeding patches on the bladder wall.

Symptoms associated with female bladder pain syndrome:

- frequent urination
- urinary urgency
- bladder pain
- chronic pelvic pain
- painful intercourse/penetration
- bloating.

Symptoms that can overlap with endometriosis:

- frequent urination
- urinary urgency
- bladder pain
- chronic pelvic pain
- painful intercourse/penetration
- bloating.

Challenges to Diagnosing and Treating Female Bladder Pain Syndrome

There is no single test that can rule out or diagnose FBPS. Often providers will suspect FBPS, rule out other conditions with similar symptoms, and then treat for FBPS. If you already have an endometriosis excision surgery planned, your provider may opt for a cystoscopy at the same time. During surgery, your provider will insert a cystoscope, a hollow tube with a lens at the end, into your bladder to evaluate your bladder wall lining and look for any signs of inflammation. But, this procedure is no longer considered the gold standard of diagnosis, with patients' symptoms being the most important hallmark for diagnosis.

It can be hard to distinguish FBPS from endometriosis of the urinary system just by sharing your symptoms with an urologist. Assessing if there are other endometriosis symptoms present and consulting with an endometriosis specialist can be helpful to get a greater insight into what could be generating your pain.

At this time there is no cure for FBPS, but there are treatments available that can help with the pain and symptoms.

To manage FBPS, you can take over the counter medications such as pain relievers, including anti-inflammatories. Some also use medications specifically designed to relieve pain and irritation in the urinary tract. Your provider can prescribe topical medications such as a lidocaine patch, vaginal and rectal diazepam, or topical amitriptyline, as well as antidepressants, antihistamines, and bladder instillations. Vaginal estrogen prescribed by your urologist or OB/GYN may also be an incredibly helpful tool in helping to reduce perceived FBPS symptoms or recurrent urinary tract infections, especially for those who may be menopausal.

Multidisciplinary care is incredibly important for FBPS patients. A nutritionist can help you avoid certain foods to improve inflammation and symptoms. Also, pelvic floor physical therapy can significantly improve many symptoms, especially urinary urgency and frequency as well as painful intercourse.

Polycystic Ovary Syndrome

I always felt like my body was a little different from my sister's. Even though I was eating the same things, I seemed to gain weight so much faster, and had a harder time losing it. I had more facial hair and struggled with acne. My mom kept saying it was because I didn't take care of myself, but I wasn't doing anything dramatically different than my sister. It was so confusing. I also had irregular periods. My provider put me on birth control to help regulate them but normalized all of the symptoms I was having. In my late twenties, a fertility specialist diagnosed me with PCOS. For years, my PCOS symptoms impacted my self-esteem, as I thought they were my fault. Little did I know I had a chronic illness that had significant impacts on my health.

–Cara, age 31

Polycystic Ovary Syndrome Defined

As defined by the patient advocacy organization, PCOS Challenge: The National Polycystic Ovary Syndrome Association, PCOS is a serious, genetic, hormone, metabolic and reproductive disorder and the leading cause of infertility in those assigned female at birth. Patients can have both endometriosis and PCOS. Providers may struggle to differentiate between the two when patients come in with challenging menstrual cycles, infertility, and ovarian cysts.

Symptoms associated with PCOS:

- irregular periods
- excess facial hair and body hair
- severe acne
- small cysts in ovaries
- insulin resistance
- weight gain
- male pattern hair loss
- chronic pelvic pain
- bloating
- infertility
- increased risk of pregnancy loss.

Symptoms that can overlap with endometriosis:

- chronic pelvic pain
- bloating
- infertility
- increased risk of pregnancy loss.

Challenges to Diagnosing and Treating Polycystic Ovary Syndrome

You or your provider may suspect PCOS based on your symptoms. Irregular ovulation, and increased androgen levels and insulin levels indicate PCOS, which can all be confirmed with blood tests. A pelvic ultrasound may also show typical ovarian cysts associated with PCOS. But, it should be noted that you can have PCOS even if you don't have all of these indicators. You can have both endometriosis and PCOS, but be aware providers sometimes misdiagnose one for the other. You'll need a well-informed provider because, while both endometriosis and PCOS patients can have ovarian cysts, endometriomas look different on scans than typical PCOS cysts.

Endometriosis and PCOS share similar challenges in diagnosis and treatment. Like endometriosis, PCOS impacts adolescents, yet diagnostic delays prevent needed treatment and care. Both diseases are often only seen as a reproductive disease, and providers overlook and don't treat the more serious impacts. If you have PCOS, you are at a greater risk for developing type 2 diabetes, cardiovascular disease, obesity, and liver disease, as well as certain other cancers. If you have endometriosis and PCOS, you are at greater risk for anxiety and depression, in no small part due to providers who miss the wide range of symptoms impacting the whole body.

There is no cure for PCOS. Instead, you must rely on multidisciplinary care to manage your symptoms. Your provider may prescribe oral contraceptives to regulate periods and medications to lower blood sugar. If you're having trouble conceiving, a reproductive endocrinologist can prescribe medications and treatments to assist with fertility. Multidisciplinary care, including nutrition and exercise, can be important tools to help patients support their health. A mental health provider may also further support patients who are struggling with PCOS.

Fibromyalgia Syndrome

> I try my best to go to my classes and keep up with my work. I am already a semester behind and don't want to graduate any later. Many of my friends graduated in May and are starting their jobs, and beginning adult life. Some days I am in so much pain and am so tired, it is hard to make it out of bed. After my fibromyalgia diagnosis, I changed my major to be able to find a job that is not too demanding, where I can work from home remotely. I am putting off graduate school for now. I am not sure what my future holds and I am just trying to take things day by day.
> –Kai, age 21

Fibromyalgia Syndrome Defined

Fibromyalgia is a chronic illness characterized by pain and tenderness in muscles and soft tissue all over the body, as well as severe fatigue. While the exact cause of it is unknown, experts think it is genetic in nature as it runs in families or can also be triggered by another health condition or stressful event. Some studies have shown that endometriosis patients may be more likely to have fibromyalgia than those without, although we need more research to understand their connection.

Symptoms associated with fibromyalgia syndrome:

- numbness and tingling in hands, feet, and face
- chronic, widespread pain
- sleep disturbances
- brain fog
- chronic fatigue
- abdominal pain
- bloating
- diarrhea
- constipation
- nausea
- headaches
- painful menstruation.

Symptoms that can overlap with endometriosis:

- chronic fatigue
- brain fog

- abdominal pain
- bloating
- diarrhea
- constipation
- nausea
- headaches
- painful menstruation.

Challenges to Diagnosing and Treating Fibromyalgia Syndrome

There is no definitive test to diagnose fibromyalgia. Instead, like with the majority of these conditions, a provider will diagnose you based on your symptoms after ruling out other causes. There is no cure for fibromyalgia. Treatment aims to manage pain and symptoms. Multidisciplinary treatment is key. Pain management, mental health support, and alternative therapies such as acupuncture and gentle yoga can help support you as well as medications that have been approved to try to treat the symptoms of fibromyalgia. Patients also benefit from stress reduction and prioritizing rest when possible.

If you have fibromyalgia *and* overlapping endometriosis symptoms, ask your provider for a referral to an endometriosis specialist. Endometriosis patients with fibromyalgia need to chat with their multidisciplinary team of endometriosis experts about additional ways to support their body through treatments.

Myalgic Encephalomyelitis/Chronic Fatigue Syndrome (ME/CFS)

It's so hard to believe that I used to be an athlete. I feel like I am a shell of my former self. There are days I am confined to bed, when even looking at my phone screen can seem too exhausting. Every day I have to make difficult choices on how to spend my very limited energy. Daily tasks like showering and eating sometimes feel like too much. I know I need to be trying to treat my endometriosis. The thought of going to pelvic floor therapy or having a surgery seems completely unattainable at this time. But my symptoms and pain from endometriosis leave me further debilitated.
   –Liv, age 32

ME/CFS Defined

ME/CFS is a serious, debilitating condition in which patients struggle with severe fatigue that is not made better through sleep and is exacerbated by any physical or mental activity. Tasks such as thinking, sitting or standing can make the fatigue worse. The cause of ME/CFS is unknown. ME/CFS seems to run in families, although we need more research on potential genetic links. ME/CFS can also be triggered by infections such as mononucleosis or COVID-19. Those who suffer with Long COVID often meet the requirements for a ME/CFS diagnosis. One study found that 1 in 3 women with CFS also had endometriosis, although we don't know the exact reason for the high concurrence rate.

Symptoms associated with ME/CFS:

- chronic fatigue
- allergies, including food and medicine reactions, and hives
- recurrent infections.

Symptoms that can overlap with endometriosis:

- chronic fatigue.

Challenges to Diagnosing and Treating ME/CFS

There are no diagnostic tests that can show ME/CFS, so providers diagnose it by taking a thorough patient history, and ruling out or treating any possible concurrent conditions. There is no cure for ME/CFS. Multidisciplinary care can help support patients in managing some symptoms, including mental health support through individual and group therapy, medical and energy management. If you have this unpredictable and long-term illness, you will probably benefit from accommodations for school or work. Just like ME/CFS, endometriosis can cause crushing fatigue. Ask your provider for a referral to an endometriosis specialist for further evaluation if you identify with any other endometriosis symptoms.

Just like with fibromyalgia, endometriosis patients with ME/CFS need to chat with their endometriosis excision expert about ways to support their body through surgery and recovery.

Hypermobile Ehlers-Danlos Syndrome (hEDS)

Having two invisible diseases that cause chronic pain has a profound impact on my life and can feel soul-crushing at times. I first got my hEDS diagnosis when I was 20. I spent many years going from doctor to doctor trying to understand why I was in constant pain. Finally, getting the hEDS diagnosis helped me understand why I felt like I was constantly injured, why it took me so long to heal, and why I was always so tired and in so much pain. I also had severe stomach issues, nausea and horrible pain with periods. Providers also attributed those symptoms to my hEDS. When I was 29 I experienced an ectopic pregnancy that required emergency surgery. It was only then that I realized I also had severe endometriosis impacting just about every organ in my abdomen.

–Alex, 41

Hypermobile Ehlers-Danlos Syndrome Defined

Hypermobile Ehlers-Danlos Syndrome is the most common of the 13 heritable connective tissue disorders under Ehlers-Danlos Syndrome. These disorders are caused by genetic changes that affect connective tissue. Each of these syndromes are distinct, with their own criteria and impact on the body. Hypermobility spectrum disorders (HSD) are also disorders that impact connective tissue. There is a correlation between hEDS and endometriosis, with a population of patients having both conditions. More research needs to be done to fully understand any connection.

Symptoms associated with hypermobile Ehlers-Danlos Syndrome:

- joint instability
- joint hypermobility
- mild skin hyperextensibility
- abnormal scarring
- chronic pain
- chronic fatigue
- gastrointestinal issues
- headaches
- dystautomina
- mast cell activation
- painful intercourse/penetration

- increased risk of pregnancy loss
- increased risk of adverse birth outcomes/complications.

Symptoms that can overlap with endometriosis:

- chronic pain
- chronic fatigue
- gastrointestinal issues
- headaches
- painful intercourse/penetration
- increased risk of pregnancy loss
- increased risk of adverse birth outcomes/complications.

Challenges to Diagnosing and Treating Hypermobile Ehlers-Danlos Syndrome

The road to diagnose and treat hEDS is very similar to that of endometriosis, in that patients face many of the same obstacles and challenges. Diagnostic delays can even be longer for hEDS as it is not on the radar of the majority of providers. Symptoms can mimic other conditions, so you are at risk for being misdiagnosed, especially because there is currently no specific test to diagnose hEDS, unlike some other connective tissue disorders. Currently, there are great efforts to understand the genetics of hEDS, with breakthroughs in research soon expected. There are also centers of excellence for EDS, but not in every city or state, creating more obstacles to diagnosis and treatment.

You will most likely be diagnosed during an appointment with an educated provider who will evaluate you according to the diagnostic criteria of hEDS. They'll take your history, do a physical examination, and rule out other conditions. Like with endometriosis, having an accurate diagnosis as soon as possible will help you avoid further complications and allow access to treatment.

There is no cure for hEDS at this time.

Pain management is an important tool if you struggle with hEDS. Physical therapy can strengthen your muscles and stabilize your joints. For hEDS patients who also have conditions such as endometriosis, which require surgery, make sure the surgical team knows about your hEDS so they can help support your body through surgery and postoperative healing, which may take more time.

Postural Orthostatic Tachycardia Syndrome (POTS)

> Historically, my POTS and endometriosis symptoms were attributed to anxiety. Friends and family labeled me as someone who was nervous, sensitive, and even hysterical. There was no amount of therapy or meditation that was fixing the long list of invasive and intrusive symptoms that made it very hard to function. It just took one knowledgeable emergency room provider to give me a suspected diagnosis of both conditions to shed light on how I had been feeling for so much of my life.
> –Corrine, age 32

POTS Defined

Postural Orthostatic Tachycardia Syndrome (POTS) is a condition in which the autonomic nervous system is not functioning optimally. The autonomic nervous system is in charge of functions in the body that we don't control, such as heart rate, blood pressure, sweating, body temperature, digestion, bladder control, and stress response. For patients with POTS, a simple movement such as standing up can cause dysregulation and a stress response from the body, leading to lightheadedness, brain fog, chest pain and palpitations.

Symptoms associated with POTS:

- palpitations
- dizziness, lightheadedness or almost fainting
- increased risk of vasovagal fainting
- exercise intolerance
- shortness of breath
- shakiness
- excessive sweating
- discoloration, coldness, or pain in extremities
- brain fog
- nausea
- gastrointestinal issues

- bladder problems
- chest pain
- chronic fatigue
- headaches.

Symptoms that can overlap with endometriosis:

- chronic fatigue
- nausea
- gastrointestinal issues
- bladder problems
- brain fog
- headaches
- shortness of breath
- chest pain.

Challenges to Diagnosing and Treating POTS

We do not know the cause of POTS, and we need more research into any genetic links. There is a higher correlation of gynecological disorders with patients with POTS, as opposed to those who do not have gynecological disorders.

You can get diagnosed with POTS after a ten-minute standing test or head-up tilt table test. Other tests such as the Valsalva maneuver or the quantitative sudomotor axon reflex test (QSART) evaluate the response of the autonomic nerves.

There is no cure for POTS, and treatments vary from individual to individual, depending on symptoms. You can take medications to help improve blood volume and blood vessel restriction, sodium retention in your kidneys, and reduce your heart rate or block the effect of adrenal hormones on your heart. You may also try gradual physical therapy with an expert physical therapist, especially aquatic therapy. Adhering to a specific POTS nutrition and fluid intake regimen may help. Avoiding certain foods, wearing compression socks, avoiding heat, or prolonged sitting, and certain postures while sleeping can also help with symptoms.

For POTS patients who have endometriosis, which require surgery, the surgical team needs to be aware of POTS. Like with hEDS, they'll need to adapt certain protocols to help support the body through surgery and postoperative healing.

Long COVID

> Having endometriosis while working as a certified nursing aide in a nursing home had always been physically and mentally demanding. The love for my patients and my desire to provide care for them helped me get through. When COVID-19 hit, much of the world shut down, but I still had patients I had to care for. The physical and emotional demands of my job felt insurmountable. COVID-19 eventually made its way to my nursing home. The grief of losing residents I cared for was just as big as the fear of getting COVID-19 and/or bringing it home to my family. I eventually did get COVID-19 and that turned into Long COVID, which I am still battling. I no longer can keep up with the physical demands of working as a CNA. My life is forever changed as I navigate multiple chronic illnesses. Taking care of my health has become a full-time job.
> –Luz, age 46

Long COVID Defined

Research has shown that patients with endometriosis are at an increased risk of developing Long COVID. Long COVID can develop after a patient has had a COVID-19 infection. With Long COVID, you experience a wide-ranging array of health problems impacting different systems in the body, which can last weeks, months or years and are often debilitating. Over 200 symptoms of Long COVID have been identified.

Symptoms associated with Long COVID:

- chronic fatigue
- joint or muscle pain
- hair loss
- gynecological symptoms
  - pelvic pain
  - changes in menstruation
- respiratory and heart symptoms
  - shortness of breath
  - heart palpitations

- chest pain
- cough
- neurological symptoms
  - brain fog
  - headaches
  - dizziness
  - change in smell or taste
- digestive symptoms
  - diarrhea
  - stomach pain
  - constipation
- increased risk for chronic kidney disease.

Symptoms that can overlap with endometriosis:

- chronic fatigue
- pelvic pain
- diarrhea
- constipation
- brain fog
- headaches
- shortness of breath
- chest pain.

Challenges to Diagnosing and Treating Long COVID

Patients face many challenges when trying to access diagnosis and treatment for Long COVID. Due to the vast amount of symptoms, providers can have trouble assessing Long Covid, especially if there are other potential chronic health issues. Many of its symptoms require care from specialty providers, leading to disjointed care. There are Long COVID clinics throughout the country, but they are not accessible to all patients and sometimes have a wait list or are at capacity.

There is no cure for Long COVID. Treatment for Long COVID requires multiple specialists, including mental health support. Treatment plans are individualized and based on your symptoms.

Mast Cell Activation Syndrome (MCAS)

I was luckily diagnosed with endometriosis as a teenager. It would be a few more years before I was also diagnosed with MCAS. All my life, I would easily develop hives. Sometimes they would even pop up around my surgical scars. I also have suffered from chronic headaches. I started taking allergy medicine every day because it helped with my headaches. If I missed a few days of that medicine, I would not only have headaches, but would get terrible diarrhea. I was away on vacation and got full body hives. I went to urgent care, and they brought up the possibility of MCAS. That started my road to diagnosis.
   –Asher, age 24

MCAS Defined

Mast cells are a normal part of your immune system. When you have an allergic reaction, they release histamine and other inflammatory agents to protect the body from harm.

MCAS is a condition in which mast cells release an overabundance of these agents, often without a clear trigger, causing a multitude of symptoms impacting different systems in the body. More research needs to be done on the cause of MCAS and why patients with MCAS often have comorbidities such as POTS, hEDS, ME/CFS, and Long COVID.

Symptoms associated with MCAS:

- chronic fatigue
- chronic pain
- diarrhea
- abdominal pain
- nausea/vomiting
- fainting
- tachycardia
- low blood pressure
- headache
- skin itching, swelling, hives
- wheezing/shortness of breath.

Symptoms that can overlap with endometriosis:
- chronic fatigue
- chronic pain
- diarrhea
- abdominal pain
- nausea/vomiting.

Challenges to Diagnosing and Treating MCAS

Providers can sometimes suspect MCAS through blood and urine tests during an MCAS episode. Often, providers will rule out other causes for symptoms, and rely on your response to treatment to diagnose MCAS. Treatment can include antihistamines and medications to try to stabilize the mast cells. There is no cure for MCAS, but treatments and identifying potential environmental or food triggers can help minimize symptoms.

Mast cells may play a part in the development and progression of endometriosis, with endometriotic lesions also releasing factors that can activate mast cells. There are overlapping symptoms of both MCAS and endometriosis and more research is needed to study their potential link. While excising endometriosis can help improve overall inflammation, if you have MCAS, it is best to chat with your provider on how best to support your body through surgery.

Autoimmune Disorders

> I try to love my body and give myself lots of grace, but some days it can be hard. Even during the times where I am doing self-care perfectly, which is exhausting in itself, my body can have a flare up. Sometimes new symptoms develop out of nowhere and I feel discouraged. One of the hardest things about having endometriosis and multiple autoimmune diseases is that I don't look sick and I don't feel sick 100% of the time. This really confuses my doctors, family, friends and coworkers. My partner understands, but I worry that one day she will be tired of it, as I know I am so tired of it!
> –Rae, 39

Autoimmune Disorders Defined

An autoimmune disorder is when the body's immune system mistakes the body's own healthy tissue as foreign, and then attacks it. According to the Autoimmune Association there are over 100 autoimmune diseases.

While endometriosis impacts the immune system, endometriosis is not an autoimmune disease because your immune system is not fighting healthy tissue; it is fighting endometriotic tissue. Research has shown there are correlations between endometriosis and some autoimmune disorders, with patients experiencing both. More research needs to be done to explore this connection.

The most common autoimmune diseases associated with endometriosis are:

Systemic lupus erythematosus (SLE)

A chronic illness where the immune system attacks many parts of the body including joints, skin, kidneys, blood cells, the brain, the heart and lungs.

Symptoms that overlap with endometriosis:

- fatigue
- chronic pain
- increased risk for infertility, pregnancy loss and complications.

Rheumatoid arthritis

A chronic illness where the immune system attacks the tissue lining the joints causing swelling, pain, inflammation, and stiffness. RA often attacks the lining of the hands, wrists, and feet, but can also impact organs such as the eyes and lungs.

Symptoms that can overlap with endometriosis:

- fatigue
- chronic pain
- an increased risk for infertility.

Celiac disease

An autoimmune disorder in which the body cannot process the protein found in gluten. When gluten is ingested, the body will produce antibodies which damage the small intestine and impact nutrient absorption.

Symptoms that can overlap with endometriosis:

- abdominal pain
- bloating
- nausea
- constipation
- diarrhea
- fatigue
- headaches
- increased risks of infertility, pregnancy loss and complications.

Multiple sclerosis

A chronic, long-term degenerative disease in which the immune system destroys myelin, the protective sheath that covers nerve cells.

Symptoms that can overlap with endometriosis:

- urinary frequency
- constipation
- painful intercourse
- chronic pain
- fatigue.

Inflammatory bowel disease (Crohn's disease and ulcerative colitis)

A chronic condition where the immune system is causing disruption throughout the gastrointestinal tract.

Symptoms that can overlap with endometriosis:

- fatigue
- diarrhea
- constipation
- bowel obstruction
- rectal bleeding
- abdominal cramps and pain.

Addison's disease

A disorder of the adrenal glands causing them to produce insufficient amounts of cortisol and aldosterone.

Symptoms that can overlap with endometriosis:

- nausea
- diarrhea
- abdominal pain
- fatigue.

Sjogren's disease

An autoimmune condition in which the glands that are responsible for producing moisture in the eyes, mouth and other parts of the body are destroyed by antibodies.

Symptoms that can overlap with endometriosis:

- fatigue
- pain.

Hashimoto's thyroiditis/Autoimmune thyroid disorder

A chronic illness where the immune system attacks and damages the thyroid gland.

Symptoms that can overlap with endometriosis:

- chronic fatigue
- constipation
- a greater risk for infertility, pregnancy loss and complications if not treated.

Challenges to Diagnosing and Treating Autoimmune Diseases

Like endometriosis, the road to an autoimmune disease diagnosis can be long and discouraging. Many times, patients look healthy to providers, even though they are struggling with challenging symptoms. Providers can see autoimmune issues as uncommon or rare, also leading to a diagnostic delay. For many of the autoimmune diseases listed above, there is no definitive testing, and symptoms can be intermittent or overlap with other conditions. Access to expert providers who are knowledgeable in autoimmune diseases can be a challenge for some as well.

Like with endometriosis, treatment for autoimmune diseases often requires multidisciplinary care. Depending on the specific disease, treatment ranges from pain management, to physical therapy, to immunosuppressant drugs, to surgery. Autoimmune conditions range in severity and you may even qualify for disability benefits depending on the disorder and its impact.

For all of these conditions, it can be extremely hard to tease out endometriosis symptoms from potential comorbidities. Through education, awareness, and collaboration, multidisciplinary providers in the chronic health, reproductive health, and expert endometriosis care communities can work together to minimize diagnostic delays and improve treatments for patients.

5
Sick and Tired of Feeling Sick and Tired and Other Mental Health Impacts

I feel scared and hopeless most of the time. I feel like a shell of my former self. Most of my friends have left me, sick of me canceling plans and always "complaining" about how I am feeling. I am having trouble working and am just waiting for my company to fire me. My family doesn't understand what I am going through and why I can't get better. With each surgery they tell me I should be fine and I just have to start being positive. But I am positive that every surgery has made me feel worse. My gynecologist said the next step is a hysterectomy, but I am only 25. He has me on this drug that makes me feel like I am in menopause. Since taking it, I have had an increase in depression and suicidal thoughts. I am still in pain. When will this end?
   —Charlee, age 25

After going through endometriosis, infertility, and recurrent pregnancy loss myself, I knew that I had to continue my work as a mental health provider in these communities. As a patient, I experienced the anxiety, hopelessness and medical trauma that other patients routinely experience. I felt bewildered that none of my providers were concerned about my mental health or even mentioned it. In fact, so many of them made my mental health worse through their practice approaches and lack of education surrounding my issues, creating more medical trauma.

During a particularly vulnerable moment, I was in so much pain, bleeding heavily due to a miscarriage after a fertility treatment. I worked up the courage to call and ask my reproductive endocrinologist if he could prescribe me a stronger, non-opioid pain reliever, as I was in a frightening amount of agony and opioids made me very nauseous. Instead of helping me, he berated me, saying that I shouldn't be in that much pain. I felt humiliated.

Later, I learned that fibroids, adenomyosis, and a lot of endometriosis were all most likely contributing to my severe pain during that preganancy loss.

One of my own patients, years later, shared a study with me that demonstrated that among women who experienced early pregnancy loss, nearly 1 in 3 showed signs of PTSD, 1 in 4 had anxiety and 1 in 10 had depression one month after the loss. Nine months later, those numbers reduced, but only slightly as women were still experiencing these mental health challenges. Often, we are not only forced to suffer in silence with our physical symptoms, but also with how these medical traumas impact our mental health.

Providers don't always know how to handle our emotions. Sometimes they aren't even equipped to refer us for further mental health support. They are often trained to suppress their own emotions when dealing with difficult and traumatic events themselves. Not all providers are trained in trauma-informed care, nor are aware of how they can contribute to our medical trauma. While they may understand on a cognitive level that endometriosis patients experience anxiety and depression, some get very uncomfortable if we express these feelings in the exam room. They deem us difficult or hysterical if we get emotional, and, as a result, we worry that if we show too much emotion, our physical symptoms won't be taken as seriously. Women are often taught to bear the burden of being uncomfortable, rather than make those around them uncomfortable or accountable. We learn it's often easier to hide our physical and emotional pain from providers, family, and friends, than share what we are going through. We are forced to package and present our pain in ways to make it more tolerable to others, with the hope we will get the care and support we desperately need.

We know that endometriosis is not only a physical illness. Endometriosis invades every space of our lives and can have a profound impact on quality of life and mental health, leading to a decrease in both. Feeling sick for the majority of our lives and not knowing when things will get better or if they will get worse is an incredibly difficult reality to adapt to. Research has shown those with endometriosis have a higher prevalence of:

- anxiety
- depression
- PTSD
- substance use disorder
- eating disorders.

While yes, chronic pain and the far reaching impacts of the disease contribute to these mental health challenges, there is research suggesting an epidemiologic and genetic association with some of these mental health conditions and endometriosis.

Unfortunately, nobody has taken any steps to transform this information into actions to educate healthcare practitioners to provide greater support for patients. We are at greater risk of chronic opioid use. Those with chronic pain, anxiety and depression are at an elevated risk of developing a substance use disorder. Flat out refusing to provide pain management to patients is not the solution. Instead, we need providers who treat us as whole people, with multidisciplinary care, including pain management and mental health support. This model of care best prevents us from developing other health challenges.

Over the years, I have worked with many endometriosis patients who are neurodivergent. Some research points to the fact that there may be a relationship between autism, endometriosis and hypermobile EDS. I also work with many patients who have been diagnosed with attention-deficit/hyperactivity disorder, which again, may have a correlation to endometriosis that needs further investigation. As an experienced provider in this field, I have learned ways to better support these patients, working with them to find tools to help them process and manage their disease. But, as always, more research and guidance is needed in these areas.

When patients have additional comorbidities, especially when that comorbidity has to do with a neurological, developmental, or psychiatric disorder, there are little to no guidelines explaining how best to serve these populations within the endometriosis community. These patients have additional struggles with diagnosis and treatment, and more challenges receiving holistic care with a collaborative, multidisciplinary team.

Anxiety and Chronic Crisis

Over the years my bowel issues, in particular my cramping and diarrhea, my severe fatigue and my horrible periods have made it really difficult to leave my house. I used to play recreational sports, date, and see my family more often. Now I just stay at home, work remotely and only leave for doctor's appointments and food shopping when I am feeling up for it. I am so lonely, but bigger than my feelings of loneliness are my feelings of fear. I fear I will never be well enough to do the things I want to do.

COVID made me even more afraid to be around others. I fear that being around other people's potential germs will make me sicker. I can't imagine being sicker than I already am. Getting on a plane seems impossible. Meeting new people seems impossible. Taking a car ride to see my sister who lives two hours away seems impossible. Spending time with my nieces and nephews who are in school and always sick, is downright terrifying. I feel like I am stuck in a very horrible version of my life that I cannot escape.

–Cameryn, age 32

For the longest time before my diagnosis, my providers blamed my endometriosis symptoms on college- and work-related anxiety. Test after test, imaging after imaging, all came back normal. Later, one "expert" endometriosis provider blamed my symptoms on the stress of being a new mom, even though he had performed an almost three-hour endometriosis excision surgery on me two years prior. I insisted that it wasn't anxiety, and another excision surgery soon after showed endometriosis had invaded my bladder wall, was causing hydronephrosis of both kidneys and also was impacting my diaphragm and bowels.

Did my anxiety cause my endometriosis to invade my bladder wall? Of course not. Yet, it is undeniable that I, like many of us that live with this disease, have experienced anxiety and chronic stress. How could we not? Living with endometriosis, especially without any support or interventions, feels like living in a state of chronic crisis. For those who have never experienced endometriosis, imagine living with a disease where your organs are fused together and stuck to your pelvic wall, constantly pulling. Imagine a disease where you don't know if you will be able to get pregnant. Imagine a disease where you are experiencing daily pain at the level that has been compared to having a heart attack. Imagine a disease where the level of fatigue feels like you have ingested twice the amount of sleeping aids prescribed, but are still required to function. Imagine a disease that impacts your relationships, your ability to work and go to school, and have an active social life. Imagine feeling nauseous all the time, or not being able to sleep because you are in too much pain and have to urinate throughout the night, or feeling like your bowel movements are trying to kill you from the inside.

Now picture everyone, including medical providers, telling you that what you are experiencing is normal, not that serious or just in your head. Gaslighting is a form of emotional abuse that causes anxiety. Despite how we are feeling, we are expected to go to family events, not miss school, grab coffee with friends, and stay late to get that work project done. These same expectations would not be placed on someone experiencing cancer, recovering from hip surgery, or even of someone who has the flu!

Because of this disconnect, we often participate in things we do not have the physical or emotional capacity for. How can we as patients not feel anxious or overwhelmed as we are forced to live in a state of unacknowledged chronic crisis? Anxiety over what others expect from us and what we expect from ourselves, despite our devastating illness, can cause us to gaslight ourselves into feeling like our disease-related challenges and shortcomings are instead indicative that we are weak in character, and unworthy of love.

Anxiety's job is to protect us from harm. Anxiety can protect us from doing things that are dangerous, such as approaching a large black bear in the wild and feeding it cookies. When we do things that we do not have the physical or emotional capacity for, we can also experience anxiety. This increase in anxiety is also our body's way of desperately trying to protect us.

A year into my fertility struggle, I received an invitation to a family member's baby shower. As the day approached, I felt increased dread and anxiety. I had my period and was in a lot of pain, and I was scheduled to have a diagnostic laparoscopy the next day. Aside from my fear of the surgery, I was also worried that people were going to ask when I was going to have a baby.

I did not have the physical or emotional capacity to go, yet *I* felt like people would get mad at me for not going. I was physically in pain during the entire event, and my heightened anxiety was making it almost impossible to sit there, as it tried to persuade me to leave the event.

When in a state of chronic crisis, our anxiety can slowly start to take control of our lives and become overzealous. Anxiety becomes obsessed with controlling the things that it can because so many things feel out of our control.

When I was very sick, anxiety caused me to stop participating in certain activities for fear that my body could not handle them, and those feelings lingered even after multidisciplinary care improved my quality of life. One time, I had to pull over due to severe right-sided ovarian pain that flared when I pressed the gas and brake pedals. After that experience, driving long distances, or on highways where there weren't a lot of rest stops, made me feel anxious. What if I had severe pain again and had to pull over? What if I urgently had diarrhea or had to urinate? Driving through mountains or on country roads with zero places to pull over became particularly terrifying as I worried about needing a rest stop. Those feelings of anxiety still lingered after my damaged and adhered right ovary was removed, and my gastrointestinal and urinary symptoms improved.

Anxiety can grow to feel so big that it impairs functioning, stopping us from thriving and reaching our goals. Anxiety can also steal joy. Outdoor activities like hiking or kayaking were definitely on my restricted activity list due to the lack of bathroom access and the worry my body couldn't handle it. While these limits seemed reasonable at first, it turned into a slippery slope as things that could even be potentially uncomfortable got added to the restrictive list as my anxiety felt more empowered. Anxiety about hiking turned into anxiety about walking in the park, which was something I loved to do. After every surgery, I would grapple with my anxiety to regain the confidence to do simple things like walk to the mailbox.

Anxiety slowly makes our world feel smaller and smaller to make us feel safer.

It can feel like a battle to make sure anxiety is not behind the wheel and driving our life decisions. When starting a clinical practice again, years after my hysterectomy and third endometriosis excision, I worried about my capacity to not use the bathroom during hour-long sessions with patients, especially during multiple sessions in a row. I had been feeling better for years, yet I was still anxious about it, and, at times, wondered if I would be able to handle it. It made no real sense; in my twenties, when my endometriosis had not yet been diagnosed and was completely out of control, I would see patients for sometimes six hours at a time without a bathroom break. Anxiety can be bossy, but often is not logical.

It can be hard to recognize when anxiety is at the wheel, especially when it is chronic. We often can feel stuck or easily triggered into a fight, flight, freeze or fawn state. When we perceive a threat, our brain signals stress hormones. Our heart rate increases, our breathing quickens, our senses sharpen, and our body tenses or trembles. We can feel this way during a pain flare, during a doctor's appointment, at a baby shower, before surgery, at the emergency room, or even during conversations with family members surrounding our illness.

When anxiety is at the wheel, and we are in this stress state, we may freeze and not be able to call the new specialist who may be able to help. We may go into a fawn state and be overly nice or agreeable to providers who are gaslighting us or obstructing care as we just want the appointment to be over sooner and without harm. We may dissociate during a baby shower because we felt like we couldn't say no to it or leave early, even though it is very triggering and emotionally painful. We may feel powerless to voice our pain during a pelvic exam and just freeze during it, tears running down our face. We are not at fault for these reactions. These are trauma responses that aim to be protective. But a good therapist can help patients be mindful of what triggers this state and how to process it when it happens, while giving us tools to try to stay present and regulated in the future.

Uncertainty is the number-one enemy of anxiety. Anxiety absolutely detests uncertainty. Unfortunately for endometriosis patients, this dynamic illness that often requires diagnosis through surgery, and may not be seen on scans, fills our lives with uncertainty.

Will I be well enough to go to prom?

Will I be able to have a baby?

Will I ever be able to have sex without it hurting?

Do I have endometriosis?

Do I have more endometriosis?

Will I have to have another surgery?

Will I be able to graduate on time?

Will I be able to do my job?

Will I ever stop being in pain?

Will I react well to the new birth control?

The questions at times feel endless and the truth is, the only thing reliable about endometriosis is how unreliable a disease it is.

We often don't know how we are going to feel, if our surgery is going to provide relief, how long we will be in pain, how the medicine is going to interact with our body, or what accommodations we are going to need to function going forward. This reality filled with uncertainty creates a lot of anxiety for patients, especially those without support or tools to help manage both the disease and the associated anxiety.

Sometimes we feel like repeating these questions or worries in our head will prepare us for things to come. If we think about it long enough and hard enough, or think through every possible terrible scenario, then we will be prepared for the worst outcome. The problem with this is that the worst-case scenario doesn't often happen. And if it did, thinking about it obsessively leading up to the event adds trauma beforehand, and doesn't mitigate the trauma during the actual event. Preparing a living will and healthcare proxy before surgery is reasonable. Having constant thoughts of dying on the operating table months before a routine surgery with a vetted surgeon is harmful. This may be anxiety's way of trying to convince you not to go through with surgery due to the fear and uncertainty of how it is going to go. In these cases, anxiety is hurting us and making things harder, more than helping us.

Diagnosing Anxiety

One way for clinicians to diagnose anxiety is through the GAD-7 anxiety scale. Through a series of statements listed below, patients share how often they have related to them. Anxiety can be scored ranging from mild to severe. When we think about endometriosis, the devastating and intrusive symptoms that come with it, including chronic pain and fatigue, along with its impact on quality of life and exposure to medical trauma, it is no wonder that, based on the below scale, anxiety is prevalent in this patient population. I have not yet treated an endometriosis patient who has not reported at least some measurable anxiety.

> *GAD-7 Anxiety Scale Questions*
> 1. Feeling nervous, anxious, or on edge
> 2. Not being able to stop or control worrying
> 3. Worrying too much about different things
> 4. Trouble relaxing
> 5. Being so restless that it is hard to sit still
> 6. Becoming easily annoyed or irritable
> 7. Feeling afraid, as if something awful might happen

Anxiety can show up in different ways for those of us with endometriosis. As a mental health provider in the endometriosis community, I support patients who experience significant anxiety. Some patients start to feel anxiety with the onset of their endometriosis symptoms. This anxiety often increases as they navigate the medical system and suffer delays in diagnosis, dismissal of symptoms, gaslighting from providers, medical trauma, obstacles to care, and an increase of symptoms that start to impact quality of life. Again, anxiety shows up in a big way to try to prevent more harm. For some patients, anxiety starts much earlier.

If you grew up with parents who have anxiety, especially untreated, you may have been raised in a culture of anxiety and are prone to the same anxious habits, negative thoughts and protective behaviors. If you were raised to say "I love you" at the end of a phone conversation, just in case you or the person you are talking to dies before your next interaction, you may have been raised in a culture of anxiety! This ingrained anxiety makes having endometriosis so much harder. Often for these patients, going under general anesthesia is completely terrifying as death seems like a very real possibility. If you were raised to mistrust doctors and western medicine in general, you are going to have more anxiety seeking out and receiving care from even a vetted endometriosis excision surgeon.

Anxiety can show up when we are little, if we are exposed to trauma or unhealthy family dynamics. When we experience childhood trauma, including sexual trauma, emotional and physical abuse, or neglect, or had a parent with an untreated mental health disorder such a narcissism or substance use disorder, anxiety may have shown up very early in childhood as a means to try to protect us from harm. Anxiety will often try to control the things we can, when faced with a difficult or traumatic situation we have no control over.

If we grew up with a highly critical parent, we often internalize that voice, and anxiety can show up as a repetitive inner critic that tells us we are not good enough and tells us things that are not helpful or kind. Endometriosis and the devastating impact it can have on every aspect of our lives can compound this existing anxiety, giving it more material to offer criticism and feelings of unworthiness. These are often things you would never say to family and friends who are struggling in the same ways you are. For those who have developed perfectionism related to anxiety, endometriosis is particularly challenging as it makes everything harder and more chaotic. At the height of my illness, I often worried that I was not enough as a wife, mom, daughter, friend and patient advocate due to all of the challenges I was experiencing and ways I felt like I was failing those around me.

Have you ever made a beautiful, elaborate dinner for guests, and then when placing it all on the table, announce that you overcooked the string beans? Or have you ever completed an incredible work project, but at the start of your presentation pointed out whatever small flaw may be a part of it to your team or boss? We can be critical of ourselves for little and big things. We berate ourselves for not meeting deadlines or goals, keeping up with chores, missing events, gaining weight, being bloated, or not exercising, even though we are in a state of chronic crisis, just trying to survive.

We keep up this stream of self-criticism while not acknowledging the ways we are strong, resilient, and competent. Never have I worked with a population so sick, yet so hard on themselves! The way that anxiety shows up often comes from trying to protect ourselves from being criticized by others. If we say it to ourselves first, we hope that when others say it to us, maybe it will hurt less. If we bully ourselves enough, maybe the things that open us up to criticism will change. But it just hurts us more.

Working with a mental health provider can absolutely help reduce anxiety. Therapy empowers us to expand our world again little by little. We learn to reframe our relentless inner critic and heal perfectionism. We start to recognize when anxiety is driving the bus, become aware of our triggers and learn ways to stay more regulated. Therapy can help us become aware of our emotional and physical capacity and put better safeguards in place to not overextend ourselves when possible to reduce our anxiety. We can also grow more tolerant of uncertainty and assess if our repetitive anxious questions and thoughts are helpful and kind or just causing us more trauma surrounding things that may or may not happen.

Chronic Grief, Depression, and Suicidal Thoughts

> I don't feel like things are ever going to be better. I have run out of options for treatments with my local provider and I cannot afford to go out of state to go to another surgeon who could maybe help. The fatigue, pain and lack of concentration made it impossible to finish my first semester at a community college. I had to stop working as a daycare worker, a job that I loved, as I couldn't physically do it anymore. My options are limited. It feels like my friends have moved on with their lives and are adulting in all of the ways that I don't think I ever will. I feel sad all of the time and spend most of my days in bed.
> –Shi, age 22

Chronic Grief: What is Lost

Endometriosis is uniquely challenging in that the disease and related symptoms can last for decades. We can feel symptoms even before the onset of menstruation and well after menopause. With no definitive cure and obstacles to expert multidisciplinary care, endometriosis can feel like it lasts a lifetime. Some patients who are able to access excellent multidisciplinary care and support may find periods of relief, or even lasting relief. But, not all of us have those opportunities or outcomes.

The American Psychological Association defines grief as the anguish experienced after significant loss. Grief also includes big feelings of regret, remorse and sorrow. Grief can contribute to:

- physiological distress
- separation anxiety
- confusion
- yearning
- repetitive dwelling on the past
- apprehension about the future.

Intense grief can become life-threatening through disruption of the immune system, self-neglect, and suicidal thoughts.

Endometriosis comes with significant loss, but unlike with the loss of a loved one, these significant losses are not isolated events, but are numerous and can feel chronic in nature, compounding over time. We lose so much to this disease. When we think about what we have lost, it is not only the loss of actual organs in our body, but the hours lost to pain, the dreams lost or deferred because of illness, the financial burden and loss due to needed healthcare and the loss of opportunities for joy and a sense of normalcy. Having endometriosis can feel like a full-time job that we never applied for, depleting our physical, emotional, and financial reserves.

What is lost to endometriosis:

- **We lose our organs.** Endometriosis patients are more at risk for losing our appendix, gallbladder, fallopian tubes, ovaries, uterus, cervix, kidneys, and parts of the bowel.

- **We lose sleep.** Some studies show that insomnia and fatigue are twice as frequent in those with endometriosis than those without.
- **We lose quality time with loved ones.** We miss parties, social events, or even just everyday moments with our immediate family because of our pain and fatigue. This may contribute to loss of relationships with friends or acquaintances. We may grieve not being able to be present for our loved ones who may need us, whether it be our aging or infirmed relatives or our children.
- **We lose financial security.** Endometriosis can negatively impact our ability to earn income and maintain employment by limiting our attendance and productivity at school and work. Endometriosis is also a huge financial burden due to the cost of expert multidisciplinary healthcare and support. Compared to people without endometriosis, we have significantly higher direct and indirect healthcare costs.
- **We lose our autonomy.** Endometriosis can put us in situations where we feel like we are stuck in undesirable or even bad situations because we do not have the physical or emotional capacity, or financial freedom to leave or change. We may feel stuck in unhealthy relationships because our spouse provides healthcare and housing, neither of which we feel like we could obtain on our own due to lack of employment. We also may feel stuck in jobs we do not like because we need health insurance and income. We may have to choose a local college we can commute to or leave our dream job because of our limitations due to health challenges. Our mobility may be impacted by endometriosis, making us feel less independent. We often feel powerless in our limited choices of treatments for the disease or choice of providers due to income, health insurance or geographical location.
- **We lose intimacy.** Endometriosis can make emotional and physical intimacy challenging in romantic relationships. Dating and building relationships with romantic partners can feel overwhelming, especially if partners in the past have not expressed empathy or support. Sexual intimacy can be painful,

leading to avoidance of sex or abandoning it altogether due to the physical pain and stressors.
- **We lose our fertility.** Endometriosis can have an impact on our fertility, limiting our family building options, including taking away the possibility of having a genetically connected child or carrying and delivering a healthy pregnancy to term. Because of the significant impact of the disease, we may not even feel like we have the capacity to parent.
- **We lose energy and parts of ourselves.** Some of us used to like to surf or ride horses. Some of us liked to travel to new places or take long car rides. We liked to cook, bake, and sometimes volunteer at a local animal shelter. These things can feel progressively harder, and then impossible to do. If we do participate in these activities, it can come at a great cost to our energy and our health. Attending certain events can require us to rest the following day or even multiple days after.
- **We lose hope.** Can we grieve hope? I think endometriosis patients grieve hope all of the time. We hope that our next surgery or medication is going to help us. We hope that a fertility treatment is going to work. We hope this pregnancy will make it. We hope that our teacher or boss will understand our absences. We hope our family will give us grace for missing the event. It's our hope, even if just a tiny sliver, that helps us put ourselves out there time and again. When things do not go as we hoped, we not only grieve the loss itself, but we grieve that part of our spirit that held positivity and bravery for a time, even when the cards felt stacked against us. Our hope reserve is not infinite, and can be depleted.

Elisabeth Kubler-Ross, in her 1969 book, *On Death and Dying*, introduced her model for the stages of grief. Over the years, critics have voiced concerns that grief comes in waves and the feelings that a person experiences are not linear. But, the feelings of denial, anger, bargaining, and depression, as it relates to grief, that she talks about are still applicable today. We experience all of these feelings related to the diagnosis of endometriosis, and all of its associated significant losses.

Before my hysterectomy for adenomyosis, I did grieve my uterus and the official end to my tumultuous family building journey, but mostly I grieved the idea of having to endure yet another surgery. I felt so angry that I was sick enough again to warrant one more operation. I tried to ignore this reality, convincing myself it wasn't that bad, as I hemorrhaged every month and writhed in pain, bedridden. I tried pelvic floor therapy, CBD oil, and other supplements to attempt to control my pain and bleeding. I stopped eating gluten, cut out caffeine and most sugars. I clearly was in denial, angry and trying to bargain my way out of needing another surgery.

Kubler-Ross talks about how acceptance is the final stage of grief. I think it is hard sometimes to use acceptance as an end goal, especially when our grief is chronic, lasting over years, and the dynamic nature of our disease and its impact on our bodies and lives are ever changing. After spending time with patients processing the denial, anger, bargaining, and depression that comes with endometriosis, I support grieving patients as they work to assimilate and adapt to the reality of their diagnosis and connected losses.

Diagnosing Depression

One way for clinicians to diagnose depression is through the Patient Health Questionnaire, PHQ-9. Through a series of statements listed below, patients can identify how often they feel markers of depression. Depression can be scored ranging from mild to severe. Just like with anxiety, when we think about endometriosis, the devastating and intrusive symptoms that come with it, including chronic pain and fatigue, along with its impact on quality of life and exposure to medical trauma, it is no wonder that based on the below scale, depression is prevalent in this patient population.

> **Patient Health Questionnaire, PHQ-9**
> 1 Little interest or pleasure in doing things
> 2 Feeling down, depressed, or hopeless
> 3 Trouble falling or staying asleep, or sleeping too much
> 4 Feeling tired or having little energy
> 5 Poor appetite or overeating
> 6 Feeling bad about yourself—or that you are a failure or have let yourself or your family down
> 7 Trouble concentrating on things, such as reading the newspaper or watching television
> 8 Moving or speaking so slowly that other people could have noticed? Or the opposite—being so fidgety or restless that you have been moving around a lot more than usual
> 9 Thoughts that you would be better off dead or of hurting yourself in some way

The Treatment Merry-Go-Round and Mental Health Impact

It's hard to talk about depression, chronic grief and its connection to endometriosis without talking about the treatment merry-go-round. The current guidelines that the majority of OB/GYNs use promote medical management of the disease. This includes prescribing drugs that may only help manage symptoms of our disease, not cure it. While we are on these drugs, the disease often progresses. The majority of providers are not trained in excision of endometriosis, especially in areas outside of the reproductive system, where much of the disease exists, leading to repeated surgeries that only do the minimum. Then, when those treatments fail, providers recommend a hysterectomy, which the guidelines state as the definitive treatment. Desperate for relief, we get this surgery, trusting our providers, only to continue to have endometriosis. After a hysterectomy, when we are still experiencing symptoms, we often have trouble getting additional care and support.

Patient advocates have fought to change the endometriosis practice guidelines to improve standards of care. We understand the physical and mental harm these guidelines cause. We have felt the loss, the anguish, the confusion, the regret, the longing, and the sadness that others face daily. With every failed treatment, we lose money, time, fertility, and hope as our quality of life diminishes. I have worked with patients who have been on the treatment merry-go-round for decades. They have spent years in pain, not being able to eat, sleep, work, or fully participate in life around them. They eventually blame themselves as providers keep telling them they are failing treatments, when really the system and guidelines set in place are failing them.

When we educate ourselves and understand the flaws in the system and the guidelines, a new layer of depression and grief descends upon us. We understand what we lost due to not having endometriosis education sooner. Acknowledging the harm that was done by previous providers due to misdiagnosis, delayed diagnosis, lack of informed consent, and incomplete and ineffective treatments is certainly part of the grieving process.

- What if we had an understanding of and access to expert care from the start?
- Maybe we wouldn't have needed that hysterectomy?
- Maybe we could have saved our kidney?
- Maybe if we got treatment in high school or early college we could have been able to go to medical school or played sports in college?
- Maybe we could have had a better shot at having a baby or would have known to freeze our eggs?

Understanding the system is set up in a way that makes multidisciplinary care inaccessible is incredibly depressing. The multidisciplinary care needed is often cost-prohibitive.

Knowing our life path and our actual physical and emotional well-being are dictated by individuals who most likely cannot even properly define endometriosis, and are part of systems that protect their own financial interests before the health of patients, is incredibly depressing. Even for those of us with access to the best endometriosis care, the treatment options often feel underwhelming, and no choice comes without hardship. Patients lament over a lack of options for treatments. We are left wondering, which of these options are least harmful and will cause the least amount of medical trauma? With the lack of research money devoted to endometriosis, we all wonder when we will have better treatment options. How about a pill that cures endometriosis, without horrendous side effects? What about a vaccine that can somehow stop the expression and progression of the disease before it starts?

Suicidal Thoughts

If you have endometriosis and have experienced suicidal thoughts, you are not alone. In the largest study of its kind, the BBC surveyed more than 13,500 women with endometriosis and around half of participants expressed they have had suicidal thoughts. I have worked with patients who are having suicidal thoughts surrounding endometriosis and the pain and other horrific symptoms it causes. Members of the LGBTQIA+ community are at a greater risk for experiencing suicidal thoughts. Every few years, the mental health impact of this disease is highlighted when the community grieves the tragic loss of a fellow patient who has died by suicide. Their bereaved families and friends share the pain and suffering their lost loved one was experiencing leading up to their devastating passing.

It is really important to know that if you are experiencing these suicidal thoughts you are not alone. These are steps to take immediately if you feel like you are in danger and need immediate support:

- If you are in the US, call or text 988, the Suicide and Crisis Lifeline, or connect on their website: https://988lifeline.org for 24/7 support.
- If you are in the UK, call the NHS on 111. There are also many helplines available; details can be found at https://www.nhs.uk/mental-health/feelings-symptoms-behaviours/behaviours/help-for-suicidal-thoughts/
- The Trevor Project offers 24/7 support for LGBTQIA+ youth: https://www.thetrevorproject.org/get-help/
- Seek a walk-in mental health clinic or make an immediate appointment with a mental health provider in your local area.

If you or a loved one is in immediate danger of dying by suicide, calling 911, or going to the nearest emergency room, may provide the urgent safety needed to prevent harm.

For those having suicidal thoughts who are not at immediate risk, connecting with a metal health provider can offer a safe space to explore those thoughts and the feelings of grief, depression and hopelessness that often comes with this disease.

Premenstrual Syndrome (PMS), Premenstrual Dysphoric Disorder (PMDD), Premenstruation Exacerbation (PME)

Many years ago, at the start of my private clinical practice focusing on reproductive health, a client came to me to help her through her PMDD symptoms. Embarrassingly enough, despite going through clinical social work school, working as a clinician at an all-girls school for many years, and being an advocate in the reproductive health space, I had never heard of it. I could see the frustration and disappointment on the client's face when I asked her more about it. The client understandably decided to seek out another provider with more experience, and I went to work trying to fill in this obvious gap in my education. I then started to question my own irritability, weepiness and big mood swings right before my period, that I had tried to manage over the years.

More research needs to be done on the potential links between endometriosis and PMS, PMDD, and PME. In my practice, I have seen many endometriosis patients who experience the symptoms of these disorders. They each have a profound impact on the patient's physical and emotional well-being, and often on the interpersonal relationships of the patients as well. The International Association for Premenstrual Disorders explains the differences between these disorders.

Premenstrual Syndrome

PMS is characterized by a set of emotional and/or physical symptoms experienced during the second half of the menstrual cycle, or luteal phase. The luteal phase is the time between ovulation and menstruation. Up to 80% of menstruators experience PMS with symptoms ranging from mild to severe. PMS can interfere with quality of life, but is more easily managed than PMDD, which requires more support. PMS symptoms subside a few days after the period begins.

Symptoms can include:

- irritability
- bloating
- breast tenderness
- increased hunger
- weepiness.

Premenstrual Dysphoric Disorder

PMDD is a cyclical hormone-based mood disorder that is included in the DSM-5. PMDD can cause severe personal, emotional, and professional harm, and even cause some patients to have suicidal thoughts and behaviors. Two to eight per cent of menstruators meet the criteria for PMDD. For those with PMDD, all symptoms subside within a few days of when the period begins.

Symptoms must include one of the following:

- mood swings: feeling suddenly sad or tearful with an increased sensitivity to rejection
- irritability: anger with increased interpersonal conflict
- depression: including feelings of hopelessness, or anxiety and feeling on edge.

Other symptoms may include:

- brain fog
- fatigue
- changes in appetite
- feeling overwhelmed
- bloating
- breast tenderness or pain.

Premenstrual Exacerbation

PME is a lesser known disorder characterized by exacerbated symptoms of previously diagnosed mood disorders during the second half of the menstrual cycle, or the luteal phase. For those with diagnosed anxiety disorders or depressive disorders, symptoms of these mood disorders may become more pronounced during this cycle phase. Suicidality, substance use disorders, eating disorders, obsessive-compulsive disorder, and schizophrenia are some of the disorders that also can be exacerbated by PME.

With endometriosis patients more vulnerable to having anxiety, depression, suicidality, eating disorders, and PTSD, premenstrual exacerbation may be a more accurate diagnosis when it comes to the emotional challenges patients experience during their luteal phase, right before their period. Pain and symptoms of endometriosis can start before your actual period begins, also impacting your mental health.

None of these diagnoses account for the excruciating pain and invasive symptoms that await us at the start of menstruation. Many of us have rituals in which we plan to do our food shopping, appointments, and busiest work days before our period. We try to plan vacations and other events around our period when we can. How can that anxiety and dread leading up to our period be categorized? It may be another factor of PME, seeing as many patients feel a lot of these sensations throughout the month. Hopefully, more targeted research, that includes endometriosis patients and others with painful menstrual disorders, will be conducted in the future.

Postpartum Depression

The period after childbirth is exhausting, overwhelming and physically and emotionally difficult as new parents adjust and recover. Postpartum depression and postpartum anxiety are medical conditions that can make this time feel insurmountable. Symptoms of postpartum depression last longer than two weeks and can impact 1 in 5 people who have given birth.

Postpartum depression is characterized by:

- feelings of irritability, anger or rage
- lack of interest in the baby
- crying and sadness
- sleep and appetite disturbances

- feelings of shame, guilt or hopelessness
- possible thoughts of harming yourself or your baby
- loss of pleasure or joy in doing things once of interest.

Several factors make us more at risk for developing postpartum depression than those without endometriosis. Black and Latina women, trans men and nonbinary parents in the endometriosis community experience more risk factors leading to the development of postpartum depression, yet are less likely to get the support they need. Other factors that are associated with endometriosis which increase the risk of postpartum depression are:

- infertility
- pregnancy loss
- pregnancy complications
- birth complications
- postpartum pain
- premature birth
- baby in the NICU
- previously diagnosed depression or anxiety
- PMS or PMDD.

Perinatal/postpartum anxiety, perinatal obsessive compulsive disorder, perinatal post-traumatic stress disorder, and perinatal/postpartum psychosis are other mental health conditions that can impact birthing people with and without endometriosis. Mental health support, including individual therapy, group support, and psychiatric support, are crucial to help us navigate these mental health challenges. OB/GYNs, pediatricians, and NICU staff are in a unique position to be mindful of potential risk factors and provide interventions, including referrals for those who may be struggling.

Eating Disorders

> I was diagnosed with an eating disorder when I was in college. I spent years in and out of therapy and inpatient treatment centers before I felt hopeful I was going to survive. When I started having my endometriosis symptoms, I went to see a functional medicine provider to see what I could do naturally to help my symptoms. I was

also struggling with infertility. Even though I put my history of having a life-threatening eating disorder on my intake paperwork, I was bombarded with assertions that the only way to fix my endometriosis was to severely restrict my eating, taking the majority of foods out of my diet. She told me that taking out all gluten, sugar, dairy and soy could cure my disease, fix my gut, and balance my hormones.

This was incredibly triggering. I had worked so hard over the years to be able to bring more foods into my diet. Feeling distressed, I immediately made appointments with my therapist and nutritionist who have helped me over the years with my eating disorder as I felt like I was spiraling into a dark place. I have since had excision surgery for endometriosis and am seeing some improvements. I also have found informed expert endometriosis multidisciplinary care providers that understand my eating disorder. I just wish that the functional medicine provider knew how harmful that consultation was.

–Fran, age 37

Eating disorders account for the second highest mortality rate of any psychiatric illness and are even more prevalent in the transgender and nonbinary communities.

Eating disorder-associated risk factors:

- biological, social and environmental factors
- physical illness
- life stressors
- anxiety
- depression
- substance use disorder
- a history of non-fatal suicide attempts.

With endometriosis, we often do not feel in control of our body. Patients report having many negative feelings towards their bodies, ranging from struggling with severe bloating, and difficulty finding comfortable clothes, to experiencing physical limitations that can come with having endometriosis. Physical activity and exercise can feel difficult, and even impossible at times. Depending on symptoms, unintentional weight loss due to nausea, diarrhea or vomiting, or weight gain due to hormonal medications or inability to partake in physical activities can feel triggering to patients. Infertility, pregnancy loss, and pregnancy complications can also create negative feelings and disconnect with one's body. We endure incredible stress while feeling powerless.

Both eating disorders and endometriosis are incredibly challenging illnesses to treat that require expert multidisciplinary care. Patient advocates in the endometriosis community have long warned that the void in access to expert multidisciplinary care and reliable education surrounding the disease has left space for influencers to promote supplements and restrictive diets as sole cures for the disease. For those of us desperate for relief, this leaves us vulnerable to develop an eating disorder based on these restrictive guidelines. Also, those who have battled an eating disorder are also more vulnerable to relapse when exposed to this approach.

At this time, no research shows that any particular diet can cure or shrink endometriosis. Actually, there is more scientific literature that supports the relationship between endometriosis and eating disorders than there is about medically necessary diets for endometriosis treatment. For some, avoiding certain foods minimizes inflammation and various symptoms for a period of time. But which foods to monitor are highly individual and best figured out with the support of a non-diet dietician who prioritizes health over weight loss and has experience in supporting patients with eating disorders. It is dangerous to tell someone who is desperate to feel better that the more they control their diet, the better they are going to feel. This creates a fear of food and adds to the anxiety they may already be feeling. Diet does not cure endometriosis and eating disorders can create even bigger health issues, and can lead to death.

Types of Eating Disorders

The National Eating Disorders Association has a comprehensive website that has support, education and resources for patients, families and providers. They define eating disorders as well as the symptoms associated with each one.

Anorexia Nervosa

A life-threatening eating disorder characterized by restricting or avoiding food intake. Many also experience a distorted body image and have the compulsion to exercise frequently. Those with anorexia nervosa may also binge-eat followed by purging and taking laxatives. People with anorexia may also have anxiety disorders, PTSD, substance use disorders, depression and other mood disorders. Patients that take medication that cause weight gain are vulnerable to developing anorexia nervosa as they try to abstain from eating to counteract the impact of the medicine.

Bulimia Nervosa

A life-threatening eating disorder characterized by recurrent episodes of binge eating followed by purging behaviors such as self-induced vomiting, laxative misuse, fasting, excessive exercise or abuse of other medications. Anxiety disorders, PTSD, substance use disorders, depression and other mood disorders, impulse control disorders, and self-injurious behaviors are all conditions known to co-occur with bulimia nervosa.

Binge Eating Disorder

A disorder characterized by repeated episodes of binge eating and eating an unusually large quantity of food in a specific period of time. Other behaviors associated with binge eating are eating past the point of feeling full, eating large amounts of food when not hungry, and having feelings of shame, guilt and depression after binge eating. Anxiety disorders, PTSD, substance use disorders, ADHD, bipolar disorder, depression and other mood disorders may also be present in those with binge-eating disorder. Patients with chronic pain are more vulnerable to using binge eating as a coping mechanism.

Avoidant Restrictive Food Intake Disorder (ARFID)

An eating disorder characterized by limiting the amount and variety of food being eaten due to several potential factors, including a lack of interest in food, food sensory sensitivities, or a fear of aversive consequences related to eating like vomiting or gastrointestinal pain. ARFID causes nutritional deficiency, medical problems and psychosocial challenges. Patients with comorbid conditions, such as medical conditions that make eating uncomfortable, as well as those with autism spectrum disorder, ADHD, and other mood disorders, may be more likely to develop ARFID.

Other Specified Feeding or Eating Disorder (OSFED)

An eating disorder where those presenting do not meet the classic diagnostic criteria of another specific eating disorder, but are still experiencing a range of symptoms.

Orthorexia

Although orthorexia isn't yet an official eating disorder according to the Diagnostic and Statistical Manual of Mental Disorders (DSM-5 TR), it is being recognized more and more as an eating disorder that has a profound impact on patients. It is characterized by a compulsion to only eat "healthy" foods in a way that is harmful to one's own well-being and health. Patients with orthorexia may also have obsessive-compulsive disorder and experience high levels of perfectionism.

Symptoms of the above eating disorders that can overlap with endometriosis:

- stomach cramps and other gastrointestinal complaints like constipation
- frequent trips to the bathroom after meals
- skips meals or takes small portions at meals due to nausea and gastrointestinal distress
- engaging in fad diets or eliminating whole food groups
- refusal to eat certain foods or cutting out large groups of food
- a compulsion to only eat foods that are healthy
- feeling distressed when safe or healthy foods will not be available
- spending hours thinking about foods that might be served at upcoming events
- a concern over food ingredients
- obsessively following diet and nutrition accounts on social media
- nausea and vomiting
- lack of appetite

- bloating
- having disturbed experience of body weight or shape
- hiding body with baggy clothes
- withdrawing from friends and social activities
- limiting social spontaneity
- difficulty concentrating
- sleep problems
- mood swings
- infertility, pregnancy loss, and pregnancy complications.

Triggers for endometriosis patients with eating disorders:

- inability to exercise due to chronic pain
- disease-related nausea and vomiting
- disease-related physical, emotional, social and financial stressors
- bloating
- the absence of a painful menstruation due to eating disorder induced amenorrhea
- fear of eating due to vomiting or gastrointestinal pain and distress
- a lack of feeling control over one's body and physical well-being
- providers recommending laxative use due to endometriosis related constipation
- providers that impart inflexible and dogmatic views on endometriosis and the curative benefits of highly restrictive diets and supplements
- providers blaming patient's endometriosis symptoms on excessive weight
- social media influencers and health coaches who instead of focusing on multidisciplinary care, promote a highly restrictive diet and supplements as curatives for endometriosis.

It is crucial for expert multidisciplinary providers in both the endometriosis and eating disorder community to work together to help support patients' physical and emotional well-being and keep them safe from harm.

PTSD and Medical Trauma

> With every medical appointment I go to, I feel a sense of absolute dread. I even started hysterically crying during my dental appointment the other day. My dentist, utterly confused, was trying to pat my shoulder and reassure me. After years of unsuccessful fertility treatments, and going two decades to doctors for endometriosis symptoms, without a diagnosis, it is really hard to put into words the harm I have experienced and what I have endured. With every cell of my body, I have a distrust of medical providers and feel panicked when I have to go to appointments, especially appointments with new providers. As someone with multiple chronic illnesses that need to be constantly managed, this is highly problematic.
> –Jay, age 42

Research has shown that endometriosis patients experience post-traumatic stress disorder more than those without endometriosis. While many, but not all endometriosis patients that come into my office have a diagnosable score on the PCL-5, a 20-item self-report measure that assesses the 20 *DSM-5* symptoms of PTSD, I have yet to meet an endometriosis patient who hasn't experienced some level of medical trauma.

So many things contribute to medical trauma which has a profound impact on our physical and mental health:

- Have you ever been in a gynecological appointment where, during your exam or procedure, the frustrated provider has told you to just relax or that what was happening shouldn't be hurting?
- Were you shamed for not agreeing with the treatment protocol the provider recommended even if it didn't align with your extensive research or didn't help in the past?
- Has your endometriosis impacted your quality of life?
- Do you feel unsupported and powerless in changing your life trajectory?
- Have you been to multiple doctors for your symptoms over the years with no answers only to find out you have severe disease?
- Did you have a hysterectomy for endometriosis only to find out that you still have the disease and that it wasn't the cure you were assured it would be?

When hearing the term "medical trauma" people often think of an unexpected, severe, or life-threatening occurrence that afflicts an individual's physical well-being. This type of trauma is often associated with PTSD. Television shows set in medical settings, like *Grey's Anatomy*, are filled with these heart-pounding moments where you are uncertain of the survival of the patient. In their book, *Managing the Psychological Impact of Medical Trauma*, authors and mental health providers, Drs. Michelle Flaum and Scott E. Hall, broaden and redefine medical trauma and its implications, for both patients and providers. Using their framework and multidisciplinary lens, it is clear that as endometriosis patients, we experience multiple levels of medical trauma that often go unrecognized by our providers and social support systems.

An ectopic pregnancy, ovarian torsion, a painful pelvic exam, miscarriage, a failing kidney, or the dismissal from a provider are just some examples of the many ways that we can experience medical trauma. I have worked with patients who experience monthly periods that feel traumatic with horrific bleeding, intense pain, violent vomiting, and severe fatigue.

Medical trauma can simply be defined as *a medical situation that brings overwhelming stress to a patient.* This definition empowers us, as patients, to decide for ourselves when we have experienced medical trauma. Patients with a history of nonmedical traumas, preexisting mental health challenges, strained support systems, and exposure to medical racism, are more vulnerable to medical trauma. But, no one is immune to experiencing medical trauma and its devastating effects.

Level 1 Medical Trauma

In her book, Flaum defines three different levels of Medical Trauma. Level 1 trauma can happen during an anticipated medical intervention or routine appointment. Endometriosis patients who have significant anxiety seeing their gynecologist, or even other providers not associated with endometriosis-related care, often experience this level of trauma. Sharing one's medical history with a new provider or even simply stepping into the waiting room of a doctor's office can cause severe anxiety for endometriosis patients, especially those of us who have been historically dismissed by the medical community. Inserting a speculum and performing a pap smear is considered routine for most gynecologists and patients, but this can be excruciating for us and feel deeply invasive on both a physical and emotional level.

How a provider handles these situations can add to or lessen the trauma you may feel. Providers who run practices deeply rooted in trauma-informed care can help alleviate medical trauma. Staff need to be aware that seemingly benign, routine procedures and appointments can be triggering for anyone. Compassion and empathy from all staff, from the person answering the phones, to the provider themselves, can help lower anxiety in a patient. Staff should also be attuned to recognize symptoms of trauma and be prepared to refer patients to a mental health provider for additional support.

Level 2 Medical Trauma

Patients experience Level 2 trauma when diagnosed with a chronic or progressive disease that can severely alter their lifestyle or threaten their lives. We live with this level of trauma, often for decades. If you also experience infertility, recurrent pregnancy loss, or other comorbidities you will most likely face additional medical trauma. PTSD, anxiety, and depression can happen as a result of living with Level 2 trauma. Flaum also explains that as patients, we can experience secondary crises when living with a chronic and/or progressive disease. Our education, vocation, relationships, and financial standing can all be significantly altered due to the impact of endometriosis.

The most successful way to mitigate medical trauma, and its impact for those with chronic illness, is to provide culturally competent, collaborative, multidisciplinary care, according to Flaum. A team approach, in a center of excellence, that can provide resources for endometriosis excision surgery, mental health support, pelvic floor therapy, fertility treatments, nutrition guidance, pain management, acupuncture, and more, would greatly benefit endometriosis patients and reduce their medical trauma. Centers that do not have a multidisciplinary care team under one roof, but offer patient referrals to resources and recognize potential medical trauma, can also be an effective model of care.

Unfortunately, this type of care is currently inaccessible to many, in part due to the lack of recognition of the complexity of endometriosis by the general medical community. Patients report that substandard care often leads to significant and repeated medical traumas, which can include repeated ineffective surgeries, dismissal of symptoms, unnecessary removal of reproductive organs, infertility, and the prescription of life-altering drugs without true informed consent.

Level 3 Medical Trauma

Finally, Level 3 trauma happens when you experience an unexpected life-threatening or life-altering event that require significant and immediate intervention. The care patients receive for a Level 3 trauma most often happens in a hospital setting.

Endometriosis is unusual in that neither patients nor providers may know how extensive the disease is until they are in surgery. A "routine" laparoscopic exploratory surgery can sometimes result in a patient waking up with fewer organs than they went in with, or the knowledge that extensive disease has been left behind because their inexperienced provider could not remove it, leading to significant medical trauma. While this does not happen to the majority of endometriosis patients, some have had a routine MRI or have gone to the emergency room and learned they have a collapsed lung, a bowel obstruction or silent kidney loss because of endometriosis. Some studies show that endometriosis patients are more at risk for ectopic pregnancies and other pregnancy complications which can be life-threatening. It should also be noted that often the level of pain that we as endometriosis patients experience feels life-threatening and that pain itself is a medical trauma.

There is a complex relationship between patients and their road to diagnosis, medical procedures, medical providers, and medical environment, with potential for medical trauma throughout. Emergency room providers and gynecological staff have the opportunity to reduce the medical trauma we experience through compassionate, educated care, while also providing further referrals and resources. Flaum explains that providers and staff who exhibit stress in front of the patient, have poor coping skills, and/or who may exhibit medical narcissism, with a failure to collaborate with other team members, can increase medical trauma for patients as opposed to de-escalating trauma.

Endometriosis patients and advocates would argue that the lack of understanding of the disease from the greater medical community, along with the outdated standards of care which contribute to the medical trauma that patients endure, makes addressing medical trauma in endometriosis patients even more challenging. Continuing to fight for changes in standards of care, pushing for disease recognition and awareness, and promoting multidisciplinary, collaborative care so patients can have an abundance of resources to navigate such a complex disease, are the only ways that we will see some relief from such a potentially traumatizing diagnosis.

6
From Harm to Hope

What Are Our Needs as Patients?

My best friend asked me what I needed to make my life better. I thought, where do I even begin? I need my insurance to cover all of my treatments for endometriosis, from out of state excision surgery to weekly pelvic floor therapy. I need unlimited sick days and flexibility at my job to work remotely. I need my doctors to understand me. I need to not be in so much pain. I need my mom to stop asking me when I'm going to settle down and have babies. I need to know that things are going to be okay.
  –Kristen, age 32

There were times, during the height of my health struggles, that the simple question from a friend or family member, "What do you need?" would make me feel overwhelmed. I had no idea how to begin to answer. So many of my needs were not being met during those times.

When our basic needs as endometriosis patients are not being met, we are in a state of physical and emotional crisis. We are fighting to survive, and thriving doesn't feel possible. If you think about other significant crises that human beings go through, like losing a loved one, getting laid off from a job, or going through a divorce, you can understand that people going through these crises often are so overwhelmed by needs, the act of delegating or advocating for one's needs as the crisis is happening is a challenge in itself. This is how many of us living with endometriosis feel on a daily basis.

Maslow's Hierarchy of Needs

In 1954, the American psychologist, Abraham Maslow, came up with an outline of needs that humans have, from basic to advanced. While there have been some criticisms of this model questioning the diversity of the humans studied, to the perceived rigidness of the hierarchy of the needs, the types of needs defined are still applicable today, especially for those of us struggling with endometriosis.

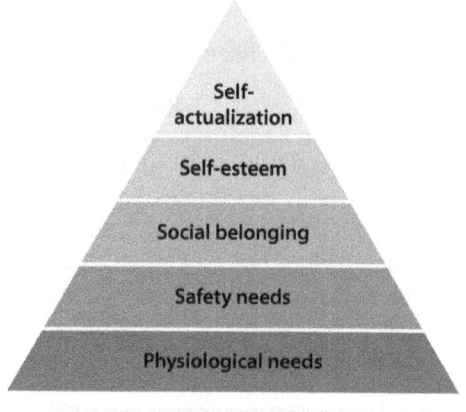

Physiological Needs

Physiological needs are foundational needs that are crucial for our survival. I often think about the 190 million endometriosis patients globally and those experiencing catastrophic hunger or those displaced due to extreme weather events or human rights violations. Endometriosis is associated with economic strain and there are patients who go without basic physiological needs who are suffering.

> **Access to food:** According to UNICEF, the United Nations agency for children, billions of individuals, largely women and residents of rural areas, do not have consistent access to nutritious, safe, and sufficient food. Food insecurity exacerbates chronic health conditions and has a profound impact on physical and emotional well-being.
> **Access to water:** According to UNICEF, at this time, billions of people around the world do not have safely managed drinking water services, lacking basic hand-washing facilities and safely

managed sanitation services. Lack of access to safe water has many devastating impacts, including impacts on reproductive health, leading to infertility, pregnancy loss, and infection.

Access to shelter: In 2023, the United States Department of Housing and Urban Development, reported those who have housing insecurity shot up by more than 12%, reaching 653,104 people. Those struggling with housing insecurity have poorer access to general healthcare, including reproductive healthcare.

Access to menstrual products: Period poverty is a term used to identify the inability to afford basic menstrual hygiene products. This issue impacts menstruators globally, leading to an additional economic burden for endometriosis patients.

Sleep: All endometriosis patients are vulnerable to changes in sleep. Research shows that we can have a lower sleep quality, including sleep disturbances and chronic fatigue. Sleep deprivation and deficiency has a profound impact on physical and emotional health and well-being.

Moving forward, a question for endometriosis patient advocates and the systems they are working to improve is how do we support the most under-resourced in our community?

Safety Needs

When your safety needs are met, you feel secure within yourself and within the world around you. While it is possible to thrive in some areas of your life without these needs being met, the absence of safety needs can make you feel like you are in crisis mode, just trying to survive. It is safe to say that every single one of us who has dealt with endometriosis has struggled with at least one safety need throughout our lifetime, with many of us struggling with multiple safety needs over the span of decades.

Health: When we feel healthy, we feel safer. Being in good health, free of disease, helps humans feel secure. Endometriosis impacts many aspects of physical health, leading us at times to feel insecure, uncertain and unsafe in our own bodies. Many of us also struggle with comorbidities. Living with these dynamic, chronic diseases makes our health feel unpredictable and unstable.

Due to the cost of healthcare and the pitfalls of getting coverage from insurance companies, many of us struggle with healthcare insecurity. Healthcare insecurity is the feeling of uncertainty surrounding the ability to obtain or sustain the multidisciplinary care we need to treat our endometriosis and support our bodies.

Employment: Employment creates financial safety and security. In some countries, employment also helps patients maintain healthcare. Endometriosis can have a profound impact on employment. Endometriosis can impair our professional lives, limiting our career choices, quality of work, ability to go to work and retain employment, career growth, promotions and bonuses. Patients also report a difficulty in maintaining a full-time job, especially a job that includes any physical exertion and has no flexibility. This lack of job security not only leads to healthcare instability, but also can impact basic physiological needs, leading to food and housing insecurity.

Protection from abuse: When humans experience abuse, it threatens our emotional and physical safety and security. Unfortunately, just about every one of us in the endometriosis community has experienced some type of abuse throughout our illness.

In the medical industrial complex, endometriosis patients are routinely exposed to medical gaslighting, medical trauma, and medical narcissism, all of which are types of emotional abuse. This leads us to feel unsafe in a system that we have to rely on for our physical well-being.

We are also subjected to actions from medical providers that cause us physical harm. Medical racism, including both implicit and explicit provider bias, has led to historical emotional and physical neglect and abuse of Black patients in the healthcare system. The LGBTQIA+ community, people with disabilities, Black, Indigenous and all People of Color are patient populations in the endometriosis community that are particularly threatened by abuse in the healthcare system.

The lack of informed consent surrounding our medical and surgical treatments leads us to agree to medical decisions that cause us more physical harm. Repeated partial and unskilled surgical interventions from providers cause us physical harm. Not utilizing proper pain management protocols during procedures, nor treating our endometriosis-related pain causes us physical harm. The difference between physical/emotional harm and physical/emotional abuse is the intent behind it. Many would argue that providers do not intend to harm us.

But, when endometriosis advocates have been telling organizations in charge that their guidelines are causing harm, and they haven't changed them, it feels more than fair to start labeling these actions as physical and emotional abuse. When we tell people they are harming us, and they continue to harm us, they are abusing us, even if that is not their intention, or they do not agree.

Environmental Needs: The environment in which we are immersed can help us feel more safe and secure or make us feel less safe and secure. For endometriosis patients, there are many ways our environment can have a profound impact on our disease.

Many of us do not live in a city or community that offers easy access to expert multidisciplinary care and do not feel safe with our local providers. If we feel scared to go to the emergency room when we are in a lot of pain, or feel like we will not get the treatment we need, we can feel unsafe. If we feel like all of our providers do not have the capacity to treat endometriosis, we can experience delays in treatment or mistreatment that leads to harm.

Living and working in safe and secure environments is an important need for all humans, but especially for endometriosis patients. Unsafe environmental factors and toxins may have a profound impact on the disease process, harming patients. Abusive environments that induce fear and constantly dysregulate our nervous systems only exacerbate our already comprised emotional and physical health.

Emotional and Social Needs

Some of the defining characteristics of humans are our social and emotional needs. It can be challenging to feel like we are thriving when these needs are not being met. Endometriosis patients are not exempt from these needs, yet the challenges we have related to our disease can make it really difficult to fulfill these needs.

Relationships: Interpersonal relationships are an important part of the human experience. Emotional intimacy in a safe relationship allows us to feel close to another person, share our thoughts and feelings, and experience empathy and validation. Feeling loved and loving others and giving and receiving affection in a platonic or romantic relationship are emotional needs that can be challenging for endometriosis patients to get met.

Endometriosis can create barriers to starting and maintaining interpersonal relationships. Our physical pain and fatigue can impede us from interacting with others. Going to family functions and social events can be quite challenging. When we are in a state of physical crisis, our capacity to be social is often one of the first things sacrificed as we go into survival mode. The anxiety and depression that can be experienced with endometriosis can also limit our capacity to form and maintain relationships, and yet the lack of interpersonal relationships can further exacerbate depression and anxiety.

Social Connection: Endometriosis has a profound impact on the social well-being of both teens and adults that struggle with the disease. It is within our nature as humans to have an innate desire to feel accepted by, connected to and in community with other humans. The physical barriers we experience going to work, going to school, attending events, and being physically in community with others, contributes to the isolation, loneliness, and disconnect that patients often struggle with.

Due to the lack of societal understanding of endometriosis, we often do not get the empathy and understanding from those we are in relationships with, causing more challenges to having our emotional and social needs met. Judgement from loved ones surrounding our disease and related dynamic physical capacity can lead us to feel unloved and forgotten by our social networks.

Self-esteem Needs

Having self-esteem is so important to our emotional well-being. When our self-esteem is intact, it can help boost our resilience when other needs are not being met. Endometriosis can have an absolutely devastating impact on our self-esteem.

Self-worth: When we have self-worth, we feel like we have inherent value. It is our internal sense that we are good enough and worthy of love and belonging. In a culture that often values achievements over character, it's easy to internalize that we are not good enough, as we sometimes struggle to meet the same achievements and milestones that our peers are meeting. Gaslighting from providers, family, friends, coworkers, social media influencers, including constant messages that we should be healthier, better, healed, cured, more productive, more fertile, thinner, in less pain, less tired, more proactive, or more accomplished, chips away at our self-worth. We slowly internalize these messages and start saying them to ourselves.

Dignity: Dignity is the inherent right to be valued, respected and treated ethically. Navigating the healthcare system over decades can erode our dignity. When the office administrator is rude to us while setting up a needed appointment, we are not being treated with dignity. When we have to keep explaining to a demeaning provider why, after our own research, we don't want to take their recommended drug therapy or go through with the medical procedure, we are not being treated with dignity. When our medical concerns, pain and symptoms are constantly invalidated and dismissed, especially during exams where we do not have clothes on, we are not being treated with dignity. When those that harm us do not take accountability, we are not being treated with dignity. This continued disrespect impacts our self-esteem.

Independence: When we feel independent, we feel like we can do things for ourselves without having to rely on other people. Having to rely on others for our physiological and safety needs due to chronic pain, fatigue, and ongoing medical treatments has an impact on our self-esteem. One of the most difficult things to adjust to, is the loss of independence over time. We feel like we are not able to do things we used to and it slowly feels like we need to rely on others more and more. For some who have become isolated due to endometriosis and are without emotional or social support, their declining independence causes high anxiety as they struggle to get their physiological and safety needs met.

Competency: Feeling competent means we feel skilled, knowledgeable and are able to accomplish things we set our minds to. Due to obstacles in accessing care, many of us feel symptoms worsening over time and our quality of life and abilities decreasing. Increased anxiety and depression can have a huge impact on our self-esteem and the ways we feel competent.

There also can be a disconnect between our intellectual or creative strengths and our physical capacity. We may take jobs that aren't stimulating or challenging because it is better for our endometriosis-related physical limitations. Over time, not using these once cherished parts of ourselves can make us feel less competent than we actually are. When we are in a physical crisis, it is hard to feel competent. Pain, fatigue and brain fog are all things that we can struggle with as endometriosis patients. Constantly battling these symptoms can have a daily impact on our feelings of competence.

Medical gaslighting, medical trauma, and medical narcissism are forms of abuse that have a devastating impact on a patient's self-esteem. Constantly feeling blamed and misunderstood has a huge impact on our self-worth. We often feel a loss of dignity as we navigate all of the challenges that come with this disease.

Self-Actualization

Self-actualization is the pinnacle of thriving. We reach self-actualization when we fulfill all that we are capable of. For endometriosis patients, this can be a tricky need to meet as our capabilities feel fluid. Our physical capacity is dynamic; we have days where we feel okay, only to be bedridden the next. Also, our physical capacity can potentially change based on what treatments we have access to and how successful they are, which is not entirely within our control. So we are forced to try to embrace uncertainty and adapt to our ever-changing reality.

A realistic perception of reality vs. denial: As a patient with endometriosis, denial was one of my favorite defense mechanisms. Being fiercely independent and determined, I did not want to "give in" to my sick body or accept help. While some in our society may have seen this character trait as a strength, I eventually recognized that I was in the denial part of grieving my disease, to my own detriment. I constantly operated way over my physical and emotional capacity, running on fumes, overextending myself to everyone around me, followed by eventual periods of crashing and burning. I was not thriving. I was constantly feeling burnt out, dysregulated and, at times, even resentful of who or what was taking my energy. The reality was my body was in crisis, and I needed to intervene to create a life that was sustainable.

Acceptance of limitations vs. constant negative self-talk: Do you bully yourself when you are already suffering? Have you ever admonished yourself for:

- Not having a clean house?
- Not getting that promotion?
- Not having enough eggs harvested during IVF retrieval?
- Not exercising enough?
- Still living at home with your parents?
- Dropping out of college?

I had to work on my own self-esteem due to endometriosis. I said mean things to myself over the years. I had to work on being gentle with myself. Sometimes, it feels like we try to shame, guilt, and bully ourselves out of having endometriosis and its symptoms. We act like if we yell at ourselves enough about how messy our car is, maybe our crushing fatigue and pain will go away, and we can just keep it clean. Maybe if we call ourselves weak and lazy, our right ovary will unstick to our bowels and we will keep being able to continue with strenuous exercise?

What if we can embrace the idea that our car is going to be perpetually messy, or it is not healthy or realistic to want the same body type we had as a high-school athlete? Our limitations don't make us bad humans. We are more than our limitations. What if we used our self-talk to love ourselves instead? How can we internalize the idea that by merely existing, we hold inherent value?

Flexibility in pursuing goals vs. feeling stuck: When we are grieving, we feel stuck. It can be hard to adapt to what we have lost and what is not possible. Before my hysterectomy for adenomyosis, I tried to start up a mental health clinical practice in North Carolina. I underestimated the time and energy it took to start my own business. Every month, I felt sick leading up to my period, and then I had seven to ten days of horrible pain and bleeding, followed by a week of severe exhaustion. It took me months to come to terms with and grieve the reality that having a clinical practice at that time was beyond my physical capacity. It was difficult to walk away without feeling like a total failure, punishing myself for the losses incurred. I ended up closing my practice, to focus more on advocacy and nonprofit work in the endometriosis space. This work was fulfilling, while also giving me the flexibility to work from home with my heating pad.

At the time, I had no idea that a few years later, after another surgery, I would be able to have a thriving mental health clinical practice. I would again have to readjust my mindset to what was possible in that moment. With endometriosis, our lives are filled with constantly readjusting to our physical capacity. We are forced to be flexible with our family building goals, our travel plans, our career goals, our exercise goals, reinventing what will satisfy our desire for growth. We have to continuously redefine what personal progress looks like.

Appreciation vs. despair: We cannot gratitude journal our way out of endometriosis, even if Aunt Nancy tells us her neighbor's sister's friend did just that. There have been so many times throughout my struggles with endometriosis, infertility, and pregnancy loss that I have felt immersed in the depths of despair. Comments from well-meaning family and friends to look at the bright side of things, propelled me further into isolation and darkness. The level of pain, fatigue, loss, coupled with the anxiety, depression and medical trauma that come with endometriosis leads to despair. When we are in despair, we are trying to survive and do not have the capacity to thrive. When despair blankets our entire life for long periods, with no relief in sight, connecting to others who have an understanding of what this all feels like, and seeking mental health support is crucial. Slowly, through grieving and processing, we can appreciate our strengths, despite our limitations and adapt to what we have, despite what we have lost.

Strong boundaries vs. subjecting oneself to harm: It is hard for anyone to thrive if they have people in their life that are causing harm, but that is particularly true for those of us with endometriosis that deal with chronic pain, fatigue and other health challenges. There are ways that we are victims to harm, including emotional, physical, or sexual abuse. There are traumas that we have experienced that we had no control over.

But, there are types of harm that we endure that we may be able to reduce if we put strong boundaries in place. Many of us have been taught that strong boundaries are selfish, that our job is to pour into others, go without meeting our own needs, feeling uncomfortable at our own expense, to uplift, comfort or preserve the ego or needs of those around us. Sacrificing our already limited time, energy, physical and mental health and well-being in these ways limits our ability to explore what we are truly capable of. When we stay with providers who invalidate us or pour energy into unsupportive family members or friends who dismiss us while demanding things from us, we experience harm. When we can put up strong boundaries with people, places, and things that steal our precious resources, we can redirect those resources into building a support team that can help us thrive.

Grieving is a huge part of self-actualization. Without grieving what is lost to endometriosis, and adapting to the reality of this disease, it is hard to move forward and create a life from what is left after the loss. Adapting takes time, like with any loss. Part of adapting is letting go of the things in our life that bring us harm, whether they are our own fixed ideas of how things should be instead of how they are, or letting go of people, places or things that are holding us back from being able to thrive.

Getting Our Needs Met: A Team Approach

After decades of trying to manage endometriosis, I finally feel like I have a team in place that I feel comfortable with. Not all of my team members are experts in endometriosis, but they all at least validate my experiences and have been open to my suggestions. While my family will never understand what I am going through, I have people in place who can be there for me in ways that my family cannot. I don't think I will ever know what it feels like to be healthy, but I definitely have more of a handle on things and feel more in control.
–Pat, 32

So often, our needs as endometriosis patients are invalidated and dismissed. We spend a lot of our precious time and energy seeking help from those around us who do not know how to meet our needs, or even acknowledge them. We try to fill in the gaps ourselves, willing this broken system to help us in meaningful ways. We often feel overlooked, overwhelmed, exhausted and discouraged.

A team approach is essential to meeting our needs as endometriosis patients. So far, when we've been talking about multidisciplinary care, we've been focusing on healthcare providers. But our team is also filled with loved ones, our extended community and society at large. We as patients are not only members of our team, we are the captain of our team and the most valuable player. Self-awareness, accountability, empathy, compassion, and trauma-informed approaches to care are essential ingredients to a successful team.

Our Inner Circle's Impact on Us

Our inner circle is incredibly important. These family members and friends have the capacity to help fulfill our needs. From emotional and social needs, to physiological and safety needs, the isolation, anxiety, and despair that we feel as endometriosis patients can be lessened when we have healthy relationships with those we love, and feel loved by. Our loved ones need to show self-awareness, accountability, empathy, and compassion in our relationships in order to be there for us in the ways that we need.

If we have a genetic relative, such as a sister, aunt, or mother, who has endometriosis, we are more at risk of having endometriosis. Our experience with endometriosis and reproductive and menstrual health, our feelings towards medicine and healthcare, and how we navigate being sick and in pain are also passed down. In our families, there are often generational beliefs and perspectives, as well as generational trauma, that can both harm and protect us.

As I continue to struggle to put together my own multidisciplinary team in my small southern city, I was complaining to my teenage daughter about an unfortunate appointment I had with my local gynecological provider who told me I no longer had endometriosis because I had a hysterectomy. My daughter looked at me and said, "What do you expect, Mom? She is not an endometriosis specialist." In that moment, I realized that I passed down the belief to her that the majority of gynecological providers do not have enough information about endometriosis to be trusted. While I am sad that this is the current state of medicine, I know this belief will protect her from some of the harm that I have gone through as a patient when I had assumed differently.

In contrast, my mother's generation as a whole were more trusting of medical providers. They were more susceptible to internalize that their endometriosis symptoms were caused by unmanaged stress and low pain tolerance, the story their providers were telling them either directly or indirectly. They were less likely to blame their providers or define their horrible experiences as medical trauma. They didn't dare talk about their experiences outside of the family, perpetuating the stigma and secrecy. Inside the family, endometriosis symptoms were often normalized. I had to find out on my own what endometriosis was, and it was only after many years of fruitless testing and medical gaslighting by providers.

In contrast, certain patient populations within the endometriosis community pass down a fear of medical providers and the medical industrial complex from generation to generation. Due to historic dismissal, physical and emotional abuse and neglect, and an increased risk of medical mortality for Black patients rooted in racism, there is a generational distrust of the healthcare system coming from generational trauma. Marginalized and minoritized patients are more likely to try alternative methods of treating endometriosis symptoms before seeking institutionalized healthcare. Other patients whose families have experienced significant medical traumas may also be afraid to get the care they need. While these generational traumas can lead to protective skepticism when it comes to receiving healthcare, it can also cause more avoidance, stress and anxiety for patients who need to seek out medical or surgical treatments for endometriosis, even with a trauma-informed, culturally competent provider.

We can ask ourselves questions to learn about our inner circle's healthcare culture and how it may impact how we approach or avoid getting our needs met as endometriosis patients.

How we grew up influences our comfortability with getting our needs met:

- How do the parental figures around us advocate for their own needs?
  - Do they ask for help when they need it?
- Was there one parental figure who always got their needs met at the expense of everyone else in the household?
- Did we grow up in an environment where our physical and emotional needs were valued and tended to?
  - Did parental figures get annoyed when we asked for help?
- Were our emotional and physical needs neglected?
  - Was it safer to stay quiet about our needs?
  - Did the adults around us even have the capacity to worry about anything outside of foundational physiological needs?

How we grew up influences how we view being sick:

- Did our family have healthcare security?
  - Did they have paid sick leave?
- Did our parental figures get annoyed or irritable when we were sick?
  - Did they try to convince us we were not sick or say it was no big deal?
- When we were feeling sick or tired, were we allowed to rest, stay home from school, or miss social or family events?
  - Were we allowed to go to the school nurse?
  - Were we allowed to miss sport practices, rehearsals or lessons when we were sick?
- Did our parental figures get annoyed if they had to come get us early from school sick?
- Did our parental figures take us to the doctor?
  - Give us medicine?
- Did they feel anxious or dysregulated when we got sick?
  - Did their anxiety and worry about us feeling sick make us feel worse?
  - Did our sickness become more about how it impacted them, more than ourselves?
- Did they just not care at all?
- Were we on our own when we were sick?
  - Did we feel unseen and unheard?

How we grew up influences our attitudes regarding healthcare and self-care:

- Do our parental figures model self-care?
  - Do they take care of their health issues and maintain their health?
  - Are they proactive regarding their health?
- Do they utilize multidisciplinary care?
- Was it okay to rest or to nap growing up?
- Was there a lot of pressure to always be productive?
- Was the importance of mental health acknowledged or talked about?
  - Are our parental figures open to mental health therapy and support?

How we grew up influences our self-esteem:

- Did we feel loved for just existing, or did we have to do things to feel loved and have value?
  - Did the love we receive from our parental figures feel conditional on our academic performance, success on a sports field or in an auditorium, our ability to get a job, or some other benchmark?
  - Did we feel more peace if we kept our needs quiet and were agreeable?
  - Did we feel more loved or valued when we put others' needs above our own?
  - Were we constantly criticized for what we didn't do, and not uplifted for who we were?
- When we couldn't perform because we were feeling sick or tired, were we supported or were we labeled lazy?
- Was there pressure to become financially successful?

Once we recognize the health culture we were raised in, and how it may have impacted us, it is easier for us to understand the ways our inner circle's healthcare perspective is harmful or helpful. This information can even shed light on what may be deterring us from advocating for our own needs as patients. Having deeper insight into the dynamics of our relationships can help us set boundaries that will protect us from harm and figure out who we can trust to help get our needs met. How our inner circle reacts to our illness has a direct impact on our emotional and even physical well-being.

Physiological Needs

There are many challenges that loved ones may face when trying to support the physiological needs of endometriosis patients. Loved ones may not have the resources to help patients with these needs, as they may be struggling themselves or just may not have the capacity.

Another challenge is that many of our loved ones don't know enough about endometriosis to know what our needs are. Meal trains, help with food shopping, help with chores and laundry or help with childcare are tasks often immediately thought of when supporting patients with other illnesses, but not always thought of during an endometriosis patient's period, or in the midst of fertility treatments. Offering to fulfill these needs or even just providing space and empathy when they talk about how hard it can be to fulfill these needs can be so helpful. If loved ones cannot lighten our load, they need to at least acknowledge our load to have a healthy relationship with us.

One of the most important physiological needs of endometriosis patients is sleep and rest. All loved ones can give this gift to patients by simply validating this need and being flexible and responsive to our request for more rest. If we say we are too tired to do something, believe us.

Safety Needs

For friends and family members, the first step in helping endometriosis patients with our safety needs is to work on their own self-awareness and emotional regulation. Leading with empathy and staying calm can help us feel safe in times of distress. When loved ones see us suffer, and they feel helpless and powerless to take that suffering away, it can trigger their own anxiety and make them feel like they too are in crisis. These big feelings may tempt loved ones to do and say things that will work to avoid, suppress, and deny the anxiety, fear, and powerlessness they are feeling, which often comes at the cost of our emotional and physical safety. Loved ones can create a toxic environment, filled with emotional abuse, in ways they may not even be aware of.

Dismissing what we believe to be our truth regarding our own health is incredibly damaging. Just before my consultation with my reproductive endocrinologist for infertility, a family member said to me, "Why does there have to be something wrong with you? You are young and healthy. You are just too stressed about getting pregnant to get pregnant. Why do you have to see a doctor?" That comment was almost 20 years ago and it still stings when I think about it. My loved one wasn't trying to be mean; she was trying to reassure me that I was okay. I don't think she wanted anything to be wrong with me, and she isn't proactive with her own health. Loved ones can create obstacles to care and emotional damage with this type of behavior.

Gaslighting from loved ones is particularly devastating. Loved ones sometimes will try to minimize or deny the severity of the illness for their own benefit. One patient I treated was feeling very sick, and yet her mom kept minimizing her symptoms to try to get her to go to an endless amount of family functions. When my patient would try to set boundaries, her mom would keep saying that endometriosis is "not that bad" compared to other illnesses. Her mom would use the patient's history of inconclusive ultrasounds and imaging to further prove her case. Her mom was an ovarian cancer survivor and would talk about how *that* was a horrible illness and how lucky my patient was that it wasn't cancer. Gaslighting is a form of emotional abuse that threatens our safety as endometriosis patients.

When loved ones use guilt as a tool to try to manipulate us into doing what they think is best, even if it is not what we feel is best for ourselves, we experience real harm. Comments like, "Your cousin Beth had a surgery for endometriosis last year like you did, but she is all better now. She just got pregnant. Why aren't you better yet? When will my grandbabies come?" are heartbreaking for us to hear. Loved ones may not think of this as emotional abuse, but inadvertently blaming us for our continued illness, and bringing up potentially triggering topics such as health and fertility, can cause anxiety, depression and further trauma. Making us feel bad about not doing things that we do not have the emotional or physical capacity for is emotionally abusive.

When loved ones are not treating their anxiety or aware of their big emotions, it can come out as anger, frustration or irritation. I had one patient who explained, "When my dad is sad, he gets angry. When he is anxious, he gets angry. When he is disappointed, he gets angry. Anger is his way of expressing all emotions. So everything about my illness makes him react in anger." Sometimes loved ones use shame to try to control the situation to make their big feelings go away. They feel like if they yell at, shame, blame, and bully us enough, they can make the endometriosis (or their big feelings surrounding our endometriosis) go away. Obviously, bullying does not make endometriosis go away, it just makes us hide our feelings or sever these unhealthy relationships. This is also a form of emotional abuse, threatening our emotional safety.

An important way loved ones can help us feel safe and prevent us from harm is by coming to medical appointments with us if we ask. When we have loved ones join us in medical appointments, and in hospital rooms, it can help in many ways. Having a regulated loved one help ask questions, record information exchanged, or request specific care is a great advocacy tool and can help us get the answers and care that we need if we are overwhelmed. Sadly, many of my patients share that when they have a loved one in the room, they get better care, especially when the endometriosis patient is female and the loved one is a male. Also, our procedures and exams can be physically and emotionally invasive and painful; having loved ones physically accompany us can make us feel safer as we navigate to and from our appointments. Sometimes we do not want or need loved ones to accompany us as we feel safer on our own, and honoring that boundary is an act of safety itself.

Emotional and Social Needs

Our inner circle plays a crucial role in fulfilling our emotional and social needs. Whether it is a platonic, romantic, or familial relationship, empathy, validation, flexibility and inclusion are the elements that we need to feel loved.

Empathy is the ability to take on another person's perspective and to be aware of and sensitive to another person's experience. Empathy enables loved ones to hold a safe space for us to talk about the challenges we are having. Empathy simply requires loved ones to listen with an open mind. Defensiveness and toxic positivity can spoil attempts at empathy. If your loved one listens to your story, and immediately shares what they are going through, centering their own needs before holding space or acknowledging what you shared, they lack empathy. If your loved one responds with suggestions on how to fix it or to look on the bright side, they lack empathy. If your loved one immediately talks about how your issues aren't that bad, they lack empathy. If your loved one shows indifference toward what you are going through or seems uninterested, that is apathy. Apathy is the antithesis to empathy.

To validate us means to affirm that our feelings, experiences and actions are acceptable and worthy. When loved ones disapprove of or question our choices, behaviors, lifestyles, and most importantly, our lived experiences with endometriosis, they make us feel invalidated and unloved. Loved ones sometimes think that if they validate our experiences with endometriosis, they are indulging us, and therefore will cause us to wallow in our illness, or give way to it. Some of our loved ones believe that if we ignore our disease and not talk about it so much, it won't have as much of an impact.

When I first started getting involved in the endometriosis and infertility advocacy community, some of my loved ones were concerned. They felt like immersing myself in this type of work would make my mental and physical health worse, and saw it almost as spiraling deeper into the disease. They didn't understand that the work that I was doing was validating and empowering. The dad of one of my patients' constantly asks her why she always goes to the doctor. He knows that she has endometriosis and many other comorbidities. The question is meant to stop her from going so much and reflects his anxiety about her well-being and his ignorance regarding what she is going through. This repeated question does not make this patient feel loved and validated.

Loved ones who want to fulfill our emotional and social needs are called to be flexible. Flexibility is the ability to adapt, change and compromise. As endometriosis patients, our bodies are often in crisis and we feel sick and fatigued. We often have to change plans, modify time spent with others, or reallocate resources dispersed. Flexibility from loved ones requires them to put aside what they need from us, so they can simply love us and respect our current emotional and physical capacity. Flexibility in a relationship looks like agreeing to order in food as opposed to meeting out for dinner. Flexibility looks like understanding if your adult child with endometriosis cannot make it to your 60th birthday party because she has her period, but instead wants to take you out to dinner when she is feeling better. Flexibility is understanding that your friend with endometriosis may need to take time away to focus on her physical and emotional needs.

If your loved one has trouble being flexible and always takes things personally, makes you feel guilty, or responds to change with anger and frustration, it can be a sign that they have their own struggles with mental health. Acknowledging their deficits, and resisting the urge to put their social and emotional needs before your own, can help you heal and find other relationships that provide the flexibility needed.

Being inclusive means to consider the needs of all of those around you, and facilitate ways that they can feel valued and included. Loved ones can create an inclusive culture for us by listening and acknowledging our needs, while not making us feel like we are a burden for having these needs. When a loved one is being inclusive it looks like not planning a family vacation the weekend following your scheduled endometriosis excision surgery. When a loved one is being inclusive, it looks like agreeing to meet at an outdoor bar because they know you worry about getting sick. Being inclusive looks like providing one or two safe food options at their holiday dinner that won't make you feel ill. There may be events that your loved ones plan that you are not up for. Maybe your loved one wants to hike for their birthday or go to a kickboxing class. Being inclusive looks like them having a conversation with you ahead of time and scheduling another time to celebrate in a way that is comfortable. When we are thought of and included, we feel loved.

Self-esteem Needs

For better, or for worse, our inner circle has a huge impact on our self-esteem. As endometriosis patients, we often have a complex relationship with our body that impacts our self-esteem. The medical gaslighting and abuse we experience in the medical industrial complex can also impact how we feel about ourselves. Our loved ones can help us fortify our self-esteem, and not further exacerbate the challenges we have.

For some loved ones, when they see us struggling, their natural instinct may be to rush in and try to rescue us. While we may need help, not letting us direct the ways in which we are receiving help takes away our autonomy and independence, reducing our self-esteem. Parents who may have co-dependent behaviors or favor enmeshed family patterns, may feel especially emboldened to take charge and "fix" everything, but that can be emotionally detrimental to the endometriosis patient who is already feeling powerless. Also, loved ones may not always know how to help and actually make things worse.

When loved ones believe in our stated capacity to be independent, and help us in the ways we advocate for, we feel more empowered. It can be confusing to loved ones, as our capacity to be independent changes, and they want to protect us from harm. When loved ones question our independence it is usually out of their own anxiety and need for control. When they express worry about us being home alone a week after surgery or going to a doctor's appointment on the train into the city by ourselves, they feel like they are protecting us. But we know what we have the capacity for at that moment. Also, we need the autonomy to learn our capacity. Going over our limits is part of understanding what our limits are. Trying to protect us from harm in a way that takes away our independence actually causes us more harm.

One of the greatest gifts a loved one can give us is to make us feel competent. We spend a lot of our lives second-guessing ourselves. When loved ones second-guess us, it profoundly reduces our self-esteem. Loved ones may feel like it is their duty to question and guide us, to protect us and make sure we are making the right decisions. Loved ones may feel anxious that if they do not assert their opinion or viewpoint, we will suffer. Say you explain to your loved one that, after a tremendous amount of research and talking with your healthcare team, you have decided to have surgery with a provider out of state. If your loved one commends you on being proactive about your health and for putting so much thought into what you need to feel better, this would make you feel competent and might boost your self-esteem. But if your loved one questions if you really need surgery, why you need to travel out of state, wondering if you really have endometriosis, asking if there is anything else you have tried to feel better, this questions your competence, negatively impacting your self-esteem.

When loved ones respect our boundaries, it helps build our self-esteem. It is important they acknowledge that we know our own physical and emotional capacity best, and they will not harm us by crossing those lines. When loved ones continuously ignore our boundaries, try to move our boundaries, or get upset by our boundaries, they are placing their own needs before our physical and emotional health. When loved ones assert what is best for us when we have asked them not to, demand our resources of time, energy and presence when we have stated we don't have the capacity, or continue to ask intrusive questions about our health after we told them it upsets us, it makes us feel small, diminishing our self-esteem.

Part of helping fulfill the self-esteem needs of endometriosis patients is to treat us with dignity. A big part of treating someone with dignity is accountability. We don't expect our loved ones to be perfect, or know exactly how to navigate endometriosis. Every day we too are learning how to navigate endometriosis. But it is important for loved ones who don't respect our boundaries, or make us feel incompetent, disrespected, invalidated, or diminished, to take accountability for their actions and to try to do better. When loved ones recognize how they have contributed to the harm we have endured, apologize, and work to do better, they are treating us with the dignity we deserve.

Self-actualization Needs

Self-actualization is often a road that we as patients need to walk ourselves. But our loved ones can help us by not casting doubt as we try to grow in this way.

Loved ones who model flexibility when it comes to our goals help support us. For instance, parents who maintain that you need to go to medical school and be a doctor may be harming you if you actually want to choose something less rigorous due to health concerns. Loved ones who put additional pressure on you and consistently inquire about family building are not modeling flexibility when it comes to their dreams and hopes for you and your capacity. Conversely, loved ones who tell you that you should not run a 5k as you might hurt yourself, is just as harmful in the same way. You may not have been able to run a 5K two years ago, but now after multidisciplinary care, you may feel up for it, even if your loved one does not acknowledge this.

It is crucial for loved ones not to get in the way of our process of adapting and accepting endometriosis and the realities that come with it. Loved ones through their own denial or toxic positivity run the risk of stinting our self-actualization process. After years of multiple pregnancy losses and failed fertility treatments, I finally decided to end my family building journey. I was grieving and trying to figure out what my life was going to look like. There were some well-intentioned loved ones that felt like now that we had given up the process, we may just get pregnant naturally. I know they were trying to give me hope, but it was disruptive to my process of trying to adapt to my new reality.

Loved ones should also try to avoid sharing any despair they feel. If your loved one seems more upset than you are about how you are doing, it could add to your feelings of despair and hopelessness. If you feel like you are more of a therapist to your loved one, and you are actively helping *them* process what *you* are going through, it takes away energy you can be using for fulfilling your own needs. Loved ones in despair about your health should seek outside support to separately process what they are feeling without being a burden.

The old saying, "If you don't have something nice to say, do not say it at all," is especially true for loved ones who are trying to fulfill your social and emotional needs. Your loved ones should ask themselves if their comments are welcomed, asked for, kind, and helpful before they say them. If the comment does not meet those requirements, it should not be said. Loved ones should always hold the perspective that this person they love is in crisis. Loved ones need to ask themselves, "How can I not further harm or stress my loved one in crisis?" and, "How can I unburden and uplift them?"

Our Illness Impact on Loved Ones

Endometriosis not only impacts us as patients, but impacts everyone in our inner circle. When we can see how our symptoms are impacting those around us, it can impact our mental health. As people with a chronic illness, we often struggle navigating our capacity to fulfill our roles as spouse, sibling, friend, child or parent.

Impact on Our Partners

Endometriosis impacts almost every aspect of our lives, and the same can be true for our partners. Our partner can be defined as a significant romantic relationship in our life that involves a long-term commitment. When not addressed, the shame and guilt we may feel about not having the physical or emotional capacity to show up in ways that our partner needs us, may cause distance in the relationship. When we are not addressing our own trauma, anxiety, depression, nor working on building up our self-esteem, it can be hard to be a healthy presence in the relationship. When we have negative feelings towards our bodies or pain with sex, it can impact our capacity for physical intimacy. If we pour into our partner in ways that we do not have the emotional or physical capacity for, it can create resentment, which in the long term can be damaging to both ourselves and the relationship. We also can feel resentful having to depend on our partner and take out our anger and frustration on them.

Partners with loved ones with endometriosis need to educate themselves about the disease. Partners who seek mental health support and community with others who understand will be more successful at providing empathy and validation for their loved one in the long-term. Communication with accountability and without defensiveness is key to a healthy relationship. When we are not able to meet our partner's needs, they may take it personally and feel unloved. Being open and honest about what needs we cannot meet and what needs we can meet within our capacity is important. Navigating challenges with physical intimacy or family building can be incredibly difficult. Couples counseling can be a great tool to help those in relationships navigate these challenges in a neutral environment. Partners need to understand and uphold our boundaries.

Impact on Our Role as Primary Caregiver

Whether as a parent to a child or cherished pet, or a person primarily responsible for a sick, elderly, or disabled family member, being responsible for another human's well-being while we are struggling with our own chronic illness can be incredibly challenging. When those we are responsible for are in crisis, we can start to feel even more overwhelmed. The daily tasks of taking loved ones to doctors' appointments, navigating school, meals, hygiene, emotional support, and social activities carries a huge mental and physical load. We often neglect our own needs, such as rest, doctors' appointments, or needed surgeries, as we don't have the support systems in place to take the time away from those dependent on us. We may feel guilty taking time away from our loved ones who need us and feel compelled to pour into them in ways we do not have the capacity for.

Finding small ways to take care of our own physical and mental health is crucial to be able to be a calm and regulated presence for those who rely on us. Exploring resources that can give us breaks and finding support services so we do not handle the weight of these responsibilities alone, can also improve our mental and physical health.

Endometriosis in Teens

As endometriosis patients, if we have a child assigned female at birth, we are more at risk for having a teen with endometriosis.

How we talk about and address the emotional and physical impact of our own struggles with endometriosis can have a huge impact on our children, but especially our teens with endometriosis. If we have a teen with endometriosis, but have never experienced the disease or chronic illness ourselves, it can be hard to know how to support them. The important question as loved ones of teens with endometriosis is, "How can we take care of their physiological and safety needs while also balancing their emotional, social, and self-esteem needs?"

Adolescence is a time of transition between childhood and adulthood. During this time, teens go through rapid physical, intellectual, emotional, and social growth and changes. Change is hard and this time can be tumultuous, filled with both literal and figurative growing pains. Teens are also under a lot of pressure from their teachers, coaches, school administrators, and their family to succeed, all the while figuring out what is next after high school. They are also under pressure socially from their peers to fit in and be accepted.

Teens with endometriosis have unique challenges as compared to adults. An important part of being a teen is individuation from one's family, and making strides to become an independent adult. Having a chronic illness can make teens feel less independent, causing stress. What can be an exciting time for a graduating teen may be filled with anxiety, as they worry about their capacity to get a job, go to college or move away from home. Things like recovering from surgery and navigating doctors' appointments, treatments and medical trauma with parents can be stressful for a teen whose ultimate goal is to spend less time with and be less dependent on their parents.

Teens with endometriosis first and foremost need an incredible amount of empathy. Not taking it personally when your grieving teen does not thank you profusely for the ways they are still dependent on you due to their illness, will help your teen process their grief.

Teens with endometriosis face school administrators, teachers, and coaches who may not understand the disease and do not provide flexibility when it comes to meeting expectations, such as attendance, performance measures, or deadlines. Often, these authority figures get angry instead of showing empathy because they do not look sick, and are assumed to have the capacity to do things they are not able to. Parents may also struggle with flexibility and empathy, like if their child has the energy to meet up with friends, hours after expressing not having the energy to clean their room. While frustrating for parents, what may be seen as manipulative on the teen's part may just be self-preservation. Connecting with friends is a crucial part of a teen's emotional well-being, and not having community can lead to negative impacts on mental health. As patients themselves, they are learning to take care of their mental and physical health, setting boundaries and prioritizing their needs.

When I found out I was pregnant with a girl, I almost immediately started worrying about whether she would have the same issues with endometriosis and infertility as I was experiencing, and like my mother experienced before me. Seeing as I could not change her genetics, I thought about what I could do to at least reduce the harm she would experience. I made sure to always talk about my infertility and endometriosis in age-appropriate ways. I always calmly and matter-of-factly explained my surgeries and my symptoms. I talked about how it was genetic, without injecting my own fear or prediction that she could have it. When it was time to talk about menstruation, I talked about what symptoms were normal, and what symptoms were concerning and could point to endometriosis. When I talked about how babies were made, I made sure to also talk about infertility and how she was made thanks to medical interventions. When I talked about sexual intimacy, I talked about how sex should not be painful. When I talked about consent, I not only talked about it surrounding sexual intimacy with a partner, but also in regards to her body and others in general, including in a medical setting.

While we cannot at this time take away the possibility of our teens having endometriosis, we can give them tools to reduce the harm they experience. We can teach them to advocate for themselves. Whether it is with their healthcare provider or English teacher, we can educate them and help give them the confidence to speak up for their needs. Part of that is empowering them to do it themselves, and assuring them that you can provide backup if they need you. When we are feeling anxious about their health or academic success, our need for control can make it hard to encourage their independence to take care of their own needs. But, helping them feel competent makes them more competent. And allowing them to be independent makes them more independent.

It's helpful to remember that teens with endometriosis may be feeling powerless, and feel a lack of control over their bodies. They may be feeling scared. They, like all endometriosis patients, are vulnerable to anxiety and depression. Seeing as the majority of healthcare providers do not even know that endometriosis impacts teens, they are particularly at risk for medical trauma, dismissal, fruitless invasive tests and procedures, and invalidation. Teens by nature have big emotions. Teens with endometriosis have a lot to feel emotional about. It can be hard for parents to stay regulated when teens are expressing their big emotions, but it is so important to hold space for their feelings.

Just like with adults, treating endometriosis in teens can look like utilizing medical management, expert excision surgery, and other multidisciplinary care. In order to reduce medical trauma for teens, it's important to find a provider that believes that endometriosis can impact teens and also has experience treating teens with endometriosis. Often providers will try to give teens oral contraceptives first to reduce symptoms. Just like with adults, taking these medications can be an emotional roller coaster for teens and so parents need to keep an eye on how they are adjusting. If your teen is going to have surgery, finding an expert endometriosis excision surgeon who is familiar with how the disease presents in teens and who is competent in making teens feel less anxious is vital. There are providers in the endometriosis community who routinely operate on teens with success and provide crucial trauma-informed care.

Even in the best of hands, teens will experience medical trauma while getting treated for endometriosis. Surgery for endometriosis can feel scary. As parents, our own fear and resistance to our teen's big feelings may tempt us to blindly assure them it is going to be okay when they express their fear. Repeatedly telling them that their feelings are silly, and it will be fine, will not make them feel better, it will make them stop sharing their feelings and make them feel like something *else* is wrong with them for feeling scared or anxious. Leaving space for them to work through their feelings will not exacerbate their feelings. Prioritizing empathy and validation, staying curious, and calmly answering any questions will help them. Also, just like adults, teens can feel isolated in having these difficult experiences. Encouraging your teen to get mental health support and connect with other teens who have had this experience can help them process their anxiety and grief.

Parents can also benefit from getting mental health support during this time. It is upsetting for any parent to see their child in pain or going through extensive surgery. If we have gone through it ourselves, it can be especially triggering as we can also experience dismay and guilt for having passed it on. As a parent, therapy can also help us process the other challenges that come with having a teen with endometriosis. It can be extremely difficult to stay calm and regulated while watching them suffer. It can also be hard to find a balance between preserving a teen's self-esteem and autonomy, while advocating for needed medical interventions they may be resistant to.

It is not enough to provide teens with the multidisciplinary tools they need, we also have to give them the foundation of seeing us utilize those same tools. What will be our legacy to our children when it comes to endometriosis?

Do we want our kids to be gentle with themselves and their bodies or do we want them to be disgusted by their bloated bellies or weight gain?

We have to model that.

Do we want our kids to prioritize rest and their health or do we want them to feel compelled to go to events when sick and in pain?

We have to prioritize our own rest and health.

Do we want them to have a supportive partner and friends that treat them with respect and help them navigate their illness?

We have to model that support.

Do we want them to have healthy boundaries with people who demand more of them than they can give?

We have to model healthy boundaries and respect their boundaries.
Do we want them to feel angry and irritable when feeling stressed or anxious or do we want them to have healthy coping tools when they feel dysregulated?

Teens by nature are learning to regulate their emotions. Anxious and depressed teens in pain have a more difficult time doing that. Shutting down their big emotions or complaints will not stop their anxiety or pain, it will just make them feel like they have to carry it on their own. Modeling being regulated and taking care of our own mental and physical health will influence your teen in the long-term, while creating a more peaceful environment.

The support loved ones offer to an endometriosis patient can make them invaluable members of the endometriosis patient's care team. Kind, calm communication and respecting boundaries are key to navigating the stress and challenges that come with endometriosis. Loved ones that are empathetic, self-aware and accountable can provide a foundation for healthy relationships.

Medical Providers and the Medical Industrial Complex

After years of going to multiple providers, spending thousands upon thousands of dollars on treatments that just led to more pain and disappointment, I finally found an expert multidisciplinary care provider who knew more about endometriosis than I did. I put tens of thousands of dollars on multiple credit cards and traveled states away to get his care. After a four hour surgery, he proudly told me he removed all of my disease.

A year and a half later, I was not feeling better. In fact, some issues felt worse. I tried calling his office, but it was hard to get a phone call back. I felt so confused as this was not the same care I had received at first. I finally scheduled a phone consultation. When it came time for the call, I waited hours to hear from him. I called the office the next day and was told an emergency came up and I would hear back from him soon.

A week later, I finally heard from him. He greeted me excitedly, asking if I was pregnant yet and then quickly became agitated when I explained that I was still in so much pain. He tried to say it was because I wasn't doing pelvic floor therapy or eating right. I explained that I was doing all of that. He told me I should get an IUD until I was ready to get pregnant and follow up with a gastroenterologist. He had nothing else to offer since he took out all of my endo.

I was heartbroken. I had trusted this surgeon and paid an obscene amount of money to see him, a debt we were still working on paying off. I feel like he treated me like the providers before him. Another surgery with a different provider revealed that I had adenomyosis and more endometriosis infiltrating my bowels.

–Jo, age 28

Are you even an endometriosis patient if you have not failed to get your needs met by a medical provider and the medical industrial complex (MIC) they operate in? Throughout my own journey with medical issues, I have been failed by the MIC more times than I have been helped. Not only has it failed to meet my needs time and time again, but its failings have come at an immeasurable cost. How can one calculate the cost of enduring decades of emotional and physical pain, losing fertility, having multiple impartial surgeries, diminished capacity to work, parent and be physically intimate, time lost around family and friends, lost self-esteem, fighting with insurance companies, time and resources spent having to keep going to doctors while being exposed to medical narcissism and gaslighting? Our self-esteem and dignity alone are priceless.

MIC refers to the health industry, which includes medical providers, hospitals, insurance companies, drug manufacturers, diagnostic and equipment companies and more. Scholars in the fields of Black studies, Disability studies, Queer studies and Feminism have examined and shed light on how the MIC continues to oppress and fail to meet the needs of marginalized communities. The health industry is a multi-billion dollar industry on which patients are dependent, by design. Long time advocates in the endometriosis community have spent decades talking about how the MIC fails to meet our needs, and how it feels like the system is designed this way, placing profits before patients.

Despite the harm built into this system, we have to rely on the players within the medical industrial complex to try to ease our suffering, while the medical industrial complex profits from our suffering. The players within the MIC know that they offer needed services that we cannot get elsewhere and set prices accordingly. There is also an immense amount of pressure on healthcare providers to provide services as efficiently as possible, which often translates to as quickly and cheaply as possible. This system not only harms us, but also creates added stress on providers that want the best for us.

Self-awareness, accountability, empathy, compassion, and trauma-informed approaches to care are essential qualities that healthcare providers and the systems they work within need to support us and prevent us from harm. Trauma-informed care at its core means, do no harm. There are six principles of trauma-informed care that aim to help patients feel safer within the MIC. They are:

1 **Safety:** Provide an environment and culture that allows patients to feel physically, emotionally, and morally safe while navigating the MIC.
2 **Trustworthiness and Transparency:** Prioritize honesty and openness when it comes to patient and provider interactions and institutional policies regarding care.
3 **Peer Support and Collaboration:** Utilize multidisciplinary care and a culture of referral to help patients meet their goals as opposed to uplifting the ego or financial interest of an individual doctor or institution.
4 **Empowerment:** Honor a patient's autonomy to make informed choices regarding their medical care and validate their lived experience. Ensure patients have power and influence over standards and policies.
5 **Humility:** Show self-awareness regarding individual and institutional strengths as well as gaps in education and ability. Take accountability for harm caused.
6 **Cultural, Historical, and Gender Issues:** Acknowledge the historical harm that has come to patients due to racism, gender, and sexual identity discrimination. Work with leaders in these marginalized communities to make medical care safer.

We can ask ourselves questions to figure out if our medical providers and other players within the MIC that we have to interact with are centering trauma-informed care and how it may impact our needs as endometriosis patients.

Are our providers and the MIC we have to navigate making us feel safe?

- Do our providers make us feel physically safe?
  - Do they explain exactly what they are going to do before they do it?
  - Do they encourage us to let them know when we are in pain or uncomfortable and do they offer pain management protocols for exams and procedures?
  - Are they gentle with examinations?
- Do they make us feel emotionally safe?
  - Do they dismiss our lived experience or shame us?
  - Do we feel like we can be emotional or share our truths without judgement or punishment?
  - Do our providers get frustrated or upset when we explain how treatments have failed us?
  - Do we feel rushed during appointments or unheard?
- Do we feel like we share similar values?
- Do we feel welcomed and respected?
- Does the supporting staff make us feel welcomed and respected?
- Do our providers and staff that we interact with show empathy?
- Does our insurance company align with us and our provider regarding the best course of treatment or are they creating obstacles to getting needed care?

Are our providers and the MIC we have to navigate trustworthy and transparent?

- Does our provider acknowledge when they don't have the information and answers to our symptoms and questions?
  - Are our providers honest about their knowledge, experience, and capacity to meet our needs?
- Are our providers able to offer full informed consent on all options for medical and surgical treatments, including options they do not provide themselves?
- Do our providers and the environments they work in offer appropriate, consistent and reliable service in a timely manner?
  - Are they able to address our urgent needs?
  - Does our provider seek out answers and referrals in a timely manner?

- Do our providers hold themselves and their staff accountable and responsible in the big and little ways they fail to meet our needs?
    - Are they prepared for our appointments, especially when they have asked for our patient history and records ahead of time?
- Does it feel like our providers and their supporting staff have a unified mission when it comes to providing services in a clear, consistent and predictable way?
- Do providers respect our boundaries when it comes to treatment?
- Are the costs and coverage of our treatments transparent?

Do our providers and the MIC we have to navigate have healthy relationships and a spirit of collaboration and peer support?

- Do our providers respect our role as the director of our own healthcare?
    - Do they empower us to make our own decisions?
- Do our providers believe in multidisciplinary care?
    - Will our providers work in conjunction with other providers on our team to ensure all of our needs are being met?
    - Will our providers refer us when they are out of their depth?
    - Are our providers respectful of other perspectives?
    - Do our providers see their peers solely as competition or will they reach out and collaborate on a difficult case?
- Do our providers attend conferences in their field to stay up to date on the latest treatments?
- Do they take an active role in understanding our comorbidities and their implications?
- Are our providers aware of programs and organizations that support their patients?
    - Do they have partnerships with these programs and organizations?
- Are our providers also advocates that fight for systemic changes?
- Do our providers seek out their own support as they navigate difficult cases and work within broken systems that make their job more challenging?

Do our providers and the MIC empower us and our choices?

- Do they have patience when they explain all of our options and answer all of our questions?
- Do our providers make us feel like we have choices?
  - Do they respect our choices?
  - If we disagree with their treatment plan or decide to get a second opinion, are they encouraging and respectful of those choices?
- Do our providers make us feel competent?
  - Do they recognize our strengths and make us feel empowered?
  - Do they provide affirmation and validation?
  - Do they provide realistic hope or despair?
- Do our insurance companies encourage us to get the best care available or the care they deem best? Are they a collaborator in our care or a gatekeeper?
- Does the patient voice hold power and influence not only in the exam room, but within the systems set up surrounding that care?
- Do patients get to share their lived experiences in meaningful ways that can lead to improvements in care?
- Are environments accessible to all, addressing any physical barriers or obstacles that are hard to navigate?
  - Are there enough safe and appropriate parking spaces?
  - Do providers present information in different ways to address any language barriers or any learning differences and needs?

Do our providers and the MIC show humility?

- Are our providers and the systems they work in self-aware of their strengths and challenges?
  - Do our providers and the systems they work in participate in critical self-reflection?
  - Are they aware of how their ego may impact care?
  - Are they aware of how their financial interests may impact care?
- Do they have a fixed mindset when it comes to treating diseases?
  - Are they lifelong learners, open to growth?

- Can our provider admit when they were wrong?
  - Can our provider apologize?
  - Do our providers get defensive when faced with complaints or conflicting information from patients?
- Do providers and the systems they work in believe in institutional accountability or do they project the institution's interests over the patient's interest?

Do our providers and the MIC actively care about cultural, historical, and gender issues?

- Do our providers recognize the historical harm that has come to patients due to racism, gender, or sexual identity discrimination?
  - Do our providers understand that this harm means it may take more time for us to trust them and the systems they work within?
- Are providers and the systems they work within aware of any potential implicit or explicit biases they have when it comes to race, gender, or sexual identity and are they actively working on eliminating those biases through education and advocacy?
- Do our providers respect our cultural norms and religious and spiritual practices when it comes to patient interactions and treatments?
  - Do our providers respect our religious traumas and strong feelings that religious ideologies should not impact our care?
- Are our providers invested in asking open-ended questions to learn more about our lived experiences?
- Do our providers ask us what our preferred language is?
  - Do our providers and the systems they work within have protocols in place to help support patients who may speak another language?

We often struggle to find providers and environments in the MIC that meet our needs. All too often, we feel dismissed, powerless and stuck in situations where our safety feels compromised. We more often experience trauma than trauma-informed care.

Providers and the MIC need to prioritize integrating the principles of trauma-informed care to reduce the medical trauma that endometriosis patients face. Patient advocates need to work with leaders in the MIC to create systems that allow patients to report medical trauma in a way that has a meaningful impact on care.

Physiological Needs

It can be hard for the most privileged person to get expert multidisciplinary care and support. Providers and the medical industrial complex are profit-driven. Those without food, water, or shelter often go without access to needed medical care. The medical industrial complex needs to work with patient advocates, organizations, and policy makers to ensure that those suffering with endometriosis who go without basic physiological needs have access to continuing care and safe places to heal from needed surgery and medical procedures.

Safety Needs

Humans who are in good health and are in nurturing environments that are free from physical and emotional abuse have their safety needs met. Simply living with endometriosis and its comorbidities can replace our feelings of safety with medical trauma. Endometriosis-related surgeries, ectopic pregnancies, bowel obstructions, and other medical emergencies cause further trauma. Providers and the MIC have the capacity to add to our trauma or reduce it, depending on how they approach care. The most important thing that providers and the MIC can do for us, as endometriosis patients, is help us feel safe, protect us from harm, and facilitate improved health.

Healthcare providers across all disciplines in medicine threaten our physical safety when they are unfamiliar with endometriosis and fail to suspect disease. Delay in diagnosis can not only cause pain and other symptoms, but harm to organ function and fertility. Taking ownership of this gap in medical education and committing to learn the basic symptoms to suspect diagnosis will reduce physical harm for patients. Providers who find endometriosis through surgery for an ectopic pregnancy or appendicitis and do not disclose it to the patient, delay diagnosis and treatment, causing harm.

OB/GYNs who are not experts in endometriosis threaten our physical safety when they attempt to treat endometriosis without having all of the tools to do so. Thirty-five-minute, incomplete endometriosis surgeries that leave disease and create more scar tissue, prescribing pharmaceutical treatments without full informed consent, failing to include multidisciplinary care in treatment plans, and removing reproductive organs to treat the disease are widely accepted treatments for endometriosis that cause us physical harm and threaten our safety. Embracing a culture of referral and sending endometriosis patients to experts in endometriosis care, will reduce the physical harm that patients experience.

Healthcare providers can reduce physical harm experienced by patients by recognizing and being sensitive to the amount of pain we are in. Pelvic exams, fertility treatments, catheter and speculum placements, IUD placements, miscarriage support, rectal exams and other treatments and procedures are uncomfortable for most, but can be excruciating for endometriosis patients. Taking extra care with endometriosis patients, especially with Black women who are more at risk for being undertreated for pain, protects us from more harm.

Providers and medical organizations are causing physical harm to patients by financially benefiting from and aligning with pharmaceutical companies in the endometriosis space and not being transparent about their potential influence and bias. Every year, pharmaceutical companies donate thousands upon thousands of dollars to the medical organizations that create standards of care for endometriosis patients. An alarming percentage of the research used to support the ACOG's current outdated endometriosis practice bulletin is funded by pharmaceutical companies. Individual providers also make a lot of money by working as scientific advisors to these companies. Pharmaceutical representatives spend a lot of time dropping off free samples of drugs to treat endometriosis to the average OB/GYN provider. While pharmaceutical treatments can be beneficial for some patients and should be presented as an option, providers must disclose any financial ties they have to these companies and fully explain the benefits and side effects of these drugs. Ethically, providers must also be vigilant about providing all treatment options along with these drugs, including referring to expert endometriosis multidisciplinary providers who will be able to give patients more options.

The medical industrial complex causes physical harm to endometriosis patients. Health insurance companies that gatekeep needed expert multidisciplinary care, hospital systems and administrators that facilitate care, and medical organizations that create standards of care for patients all inflict physical and emotional harm on us. Failing to adequately define the disease, recognize it as a complex subspecialty, and work with multidisciplinary experts and patient advocates to create accurate and culturally competent education and standards of care to address delays in diagnosis, misdiagnoses and deficient care harms us.

Emotional and Social Needs

Medical providers and the medical industrial complex can reduce emotional harm by providing culturally competent care to the most marginalized in the endometriosis community. Anti-racism training for all of those who interact with patients, including exploring explicit and implicit bias along with historical and systemic racism in medical care, will reduce harm and provide emotional and physical safety for impacted patients. Focusing on health equity for endometriosis patients will reduce physical and emotional harm.

Trauma-informed care addresses the systems and narratives that discriminate against race, gender, sexual identity, culture, and spiritual beliefs. Leaving space for and affirming a patient's pronouns or romantic partner, providing care for patients that is directed by their own personal beliefs and values, and finding ways to culturally translate care for those in need, are ways to help patients feel emotionally safe and reduce trauma.

Medical narcissism afflicts both individual providers and the medical industrial complex as a whole, causing great emotional harm to patients. In his book, *Medical Errors and Medical Narcissism*, author John Banja defines narcissism as a psychological defense that protects against uncomfortable challenges to a person's sense of self. While not all individual providers fit the criteria to be diagnosed as having narcissistic personality disorder according to the DSM-5, some may fit that criteria, and others may display behavior that belongs on the spectrum of medical narcissism.

John Banja provides clues as to whether or not your provider may be exhibiting medical narcissism. Your provider may be displaying medical narcissism if they lack empathy and do not react to your grief, pain or suffering. Big emotions may make providers feel anxious or uncomfortable. Instead of displaying empathy or patient-centered behavior, they may respond with apathy, anger, or self-protective behavior. This looks like avoiding admitting to making mistakes, having to always be perceived as competent, never admitting ignorance, displaying rigidity with care, and preferring patients who are submissive and do not question them.

Your provider may be displaying symptoms of medical narcissism if they cannot tolerate your lack of progress. Endometriosis is incredibly difficult to treat and may threaten the ego of a provider who is a perfectionist and sees your success as defining whether they are good or bad at their job. If you make them feel like they are incompetent or inadequate at their job, they may dismiss you, lash out at you, blame you for your lack of progress or positive outcome. If your case is challenging or makes them feel like a failure, they may distance themselves from you or release you as a patient in a way that provides no explanation or closure. Dismissal and blaming the patient for their continued pain is medical gaslighting that is a form of emotional abuse.

Other providers who experience extreme medical narcissism may take full credit for your successes and try to exploit your medical history for their own benefit. They often exhibit a savior complex, craving constant affirmation that they are superior. These providers may be gifted, but their arrogance and need for constant praise and gratitude from patients and the community at large is indicative of how emotionally fragile they are. These providers are often controlling and lash out at patients when they want a second opinion or advocate for a different treatment plan than the one being recommended.

Medical narcissism is baked into the medical industrial complex. Healthcare insurance companies and medical organizations hold power over care and treatments and are financially motivated to hold onto that power. Endometriosis patients have spent decades presenting their pain and suffering, lack of access to care, and harm that they have endured at the hands of poor policies and standards of care, and yet, nothing changes. Institutional leaders continue to deny us access to expert multidisciplinary care, updated standards of care and better medical education. This demonstrates a systemic lack of empathy, a rigid need to control care, and a universal refusal to admit widespread incompetence and inadequacy in care. As long as these standards stay in place, providers will continue to feel emboldened to provide poor quality care and patients will not have grounds to take legal action for harmful care.

Not harming us is the bare minimum requirement for providers and the MIC. We have emotional and social needs that can also be filled by the medical community.

Providers and the MIC need to understand the emotional and social implications of endometriosis and how truly devastating a disease it is. We, as patients, don't only need a competent medical system, we need all parties involved to validate our lived experience and show us empathy at every turn. We need openness and flexibility when it comes to our care. If a provider cannot treat our disease, they should validate our experience and refer us to someone else who will help. Providers and health insurance companies also have to be mindful of the impact endometriosis has on mental health and have referrals on hand for mental health support.

When patients are diagnosed with cancer, they are often given referrals to groups and community organizations that can provide further support and resources. There is an acknowledgement that this is too big of a diagnosis to tackle alone. Providers have an opportunity to partner with endometriosis organizations and advocates to share information regarding social meetups and support groups.

Self-esteem Needs

Paternalism in medicine impacts the self-esteem of patients. When an insurance company denies care from a specialist or makes us fail numerous treatments before approving the one we know we need, it robs us not only of our health, but of our autonomy. When a provider blames our endometriosis symptoms on our weight or diet, insists that we have failed treatments instead of treatments failing us, or denies our request for a referral, it impacts our dignity and makes us feel less competent. Providers instead need to empower us and believe in our capacity to make our own healthcare decisions based on our understanding of our lived experiences and our goals.

Fostering a culture of atonement among providers and the medical industrial complex would also help the self-esteem needs of patients. Providers who miss the diagnosis or perform an incomplete surgery have the opportunity to make amends with their patients by admitting this fact and apologizing for it. We have been historically dismissed and mistreated. We have been gaslighted and made to feel powerless and hysterical. Forging new standards of care with patient advocates and recognizing the harm done would go a long way to help us heal from these medical traumas. Until widespread accountability for these transgressions happens, it will be hard for us patients to trust providers and the medical industrial complex as a whole. Constantly having to rely on this broken system impacts our self-esteem.

Self-actualization Needs

Providers can help patients adapt to their endometriosis diagnosis through education and transparency. When providers have a deep understanding of endometriosis and all that comes with it, we can start to process the reality of living with the disease. Being transparent regarding medical treatments, surgical findings and outcomes can also help us adapt to our diagnosis. Providing comprehensive case notes, surgical notes, pictures, and videos can also help us adapt to our diagnosis and get continued care.

Treating endometriosis is overwhelming and frustrating for many providers, but it is crucial that providers understand that it is our feelings of frustration and being overwhelmed that need to be centered in the patient-provider relationship. For providers who may not understand endometriosis, divulging their own strengths and limitations, and referring out to multidisciplinary experts, can help us feel less despair. If providers are feeling vulnerable, powerless, or in despair regarding our healthcare, they need to seek out mental health support and collaborate with other providers in the field so as not to put those feelings on us. As patients, we appreciate if providers are honest regarding the challenges of treating endometriosis, but if we get the sense that our providers are in despair, it can cause us to panic. Providers need to stay emotionally regulated as they validate our big feelings and emotions surrounding our illness.

How Can Society, Employers and Our Government Work With Us to Fulfill Our Needs?

Seeing the road blocks my teenage daughter is facing, not only due to her endometriosis, but due to the lack of societal understanding and institutional support is very disheartening. Her teachers and school administrators have not been understanding nor supportive when it has come to her endometriosis-related absences. Her school allows ten absences a semester, and every semester she has easily run through those absences. Sometimes she has a doctor's note, like when she had her excision surgery, which has excused her absences, but she doesn't go to the doctor every time her period is painful and heavy. Even though she has kept straight As and makes up all of her work, I still worry they will not let her pass each semester because of their absence policy.

My daughter doesn't qualify for extra time on standardized tests, even though when she is in pain, it impacts her ability to think and takes her more time. Her ACT fell on her period, and she came home crying because she couldn't finish and was in so much pain. There are scholarships that seniors in high school can apply for that cater to almost every illness and disease out there, but none for endometriosis. In college, I have heard that some professors are even less flexible about absences. I am worried that the lack of flexibility set up by the institutions around her will limit her capacity to succeed in the ways I know she could if she just had more empathy and understanding.
–Karin, age 46

Our academic institutions, employers, governments, and societies at large can meet our needs by embracing our disease and the culture of empathy that we ask of our loved ones and healthcare providers. Currently, it feels like these entities are failing us and even adding to our trauma when they have the capacity to provide interventions to prevent us from experiencing more harm, but do not act on them.

Patient advocates and their allies have been working for decades to improve awareness and empathy for endometriosis because, despite its prevalence, many people have never heard of it. For other diseases and health challenges throughout history, public health leaders and organizations, with the input of patient advocates, have identified the health problems at hand, and worked to create solutions to improve health outcomes. However, endometriosis faces unique challenges in getting the same widespread awareness and support.

The stigmas surrounding reproductive and menstrual health have created obstacles to gathering societal and political support. Endometriosis is hard for patients to talk about, partially because when menstruators start talking about their period, those listening may find it off-putting, especially men. Many adults disagree on how to educate adolescents on this topic, which falls under the umbrella of reproductive and sexual health. Some believe that we should restrict education or provide no education at all. When our society at large or our politicians do not know what a fallopian tube is or how menstruation works, there is more ground to cover when trying to rally support for a disease that has been centered around painful periods. Patient advocates have long said the key to gaining more support and awareness is to reframe the current view of endometriosis from being a menstrual disease to what it really is, a full body disease, as it impacts multiple systems in the body.

Over the years, much of the awareness created surrounding endometriosis has not been accurate. Well-intentioned celebrities who have spoken about their experience with endometriosis define endometriosis inaccurately or talk about how a hysterectomy saved them. Sometimes their stories uplift their specific surgeon, acting more like an advertisement rather than a call for social action. During endometriosis awareness month in March, more and more articles tout inaccurate information. Journalists interview the average OB/GYN, a self-proclaimed OB/GYN, "endometriosis expert" who, further spreads misinformation. Pharmaceutical companies roll out ads for their products, disguised as endometriosis awareness campaigns. Journalists have published articles on endometriosis in which they interview paid medical advisors from pharmaceutical companies, often without disclosing their affiliation and potential bias. These articles not only read like pharma ads but sometimes even contain actual pharma ads.

Endometriosis historically has been under-researched and underfunded compared to other diseases that have a lesser prevalence like Crohn's disease or rheumatoid arthritis. Advocates have rightly inferred that, because endometriosis primarily impacts women and those assigned female at birth, and is associated with menstruation and chronic pain, it is not given the same attention and funds as diseases that hold the same socioeconomic burden with less prevalence. Over the years patient advocates have fought to get more funding through political and social support, but more is desperately needed.

Governments at the local, state and federal level have the opportunity to help fulfill the needs of endometriosis patients. When politicians have endometriosis, themselves, or have a family member or constituent with endometriosis, this can inspire them to act. These politicians then work to find allies and garner support to implement policies and allocate resources that benefit endometriosis patients. Throughout history, the federal government's role in supporting state and local health agencies, policies, services, and initiatives has changed based on the political and social values of the time. Restrictive policies based on political or religious beliefs, such as restricting life-saving intervention for ectopic pregnancies, are made without empathy for, or medical knowledge of, what we go through. These policies not only fail to meet our needs, they actively harm us and cause us more medical trauma.

In thinking about our relationship with employers, I often think about the phrase, "Cut off your nose to spite your face." The inflexibility given to employees, when there is a capacity to be flexible, the expensive and often restrictive healthcare offered, the toxic work cultures that don't promote work-life balance, and the value of profit over the people who are creating the profit, ultimately lends itself to productivity loss and employee burnout. These environments are harmful to all humans, but especially destructive to the emotional and physical health of endometriosis patients.

Academic institutions have a unique opportunity to help fulfill the needs of students with endometriosis. Flexibility in regards to absences and remote learning, endometriosis awareness among teachers and administrators, and educated school nurses and school counselors regarding signs and symptoms of endometriosis are some of the ways that students with endometriosis can feel supported within their academic institutions.

Endometriosis patient advocates have worked hard over the years to build bridges with interested parties throughout society, government, employers, and schools to improve the well-being of those in the community. The initiatives that have sparked change and movement are diverse in nature:

- Globally premiered documentaries, such as filmmaker Shannon Cohn's *Below the Belt*, whose bipartisan advocacy work also led to increased funding for endometriosis through the Department of Defense.
- Adolescent education programs, such as the groundbreaking MISE (Menstrual Information Specialising in Endometriosis) Program in Ireland, working to educate young people on endometriosis and menstrual health.
- EndoRise, an initiative to advance endometriosis research, awareness and education in the state of Connecticut, created by the Endometriosis Working Group in collaboration with state legislators and other interested parties.
- Research studies, such as those led by George Mason University College of Public Health in collaboration with Lauren Kornegay, the Founder and Executive Director of the nonprofit Endo Black, Inc., focused on historically underserved populations in the endometriosis community.
  - Dr. Jhumka Gupta is working with Ms. Kornegay on SurrEndo, a federally funded research study using gaming to reduce stigma among Black and Latina adolescents/young women with endometriosis or suspected endometriosis.

- Doctoral candidate, Julia Mandeville, along with Drs. Anna Pollack and Jhumka Gupta, are working with Ms. Kornegay on ENDO-served, a study which aims to understand the social and healthcare experiences of Black women and other women of color who have endometriosis.

All of the most impactful initiatives are led by patients and have the same overarching goals to improve the lives of patients.

Examples of Goals for Societal Interventions

1 **Perpetuate patient-led awareness and education.** These should be transparent and unbiased, correctly citing endometriosis as a physically and emotionally devastating, lifelong, incurable, multisystemic disease that requires expert, multidisciplinary care.
2 **Reduce the stigma.** Continue to learn and talk about sexual and reproductive health.
3 **Work with current thought leaders and nonprofits in public health.** Seek out conversations, especially in the reproductive health, infertility, and chronic illness spaces to be more inclusive of the needs of endometriosis patients in their mission, particularly those most minoritized and marginalized in our community, to improve health inequities which lead to healthcare disparities.

Examples of Goals for Government-driven Interventions

1 **Recognize endometriosis as a disability.** Because endometriosis isn't recognized as a disability, patients with housing, healthcare and food insecurity often do not qualify for the same support as others with comparable health challenges. Autoimmune diseases and inflammatory bowel diseases are some of the chronic illnesses that do qualify. Allowing patients with endometriosis the option to qualify for disability benefits would be life-changing for so many.
2 **Protect diversity, equity and inclusion initiatives.** Local, state and federal governments can help with the safety needs

of endometriosis patients in many ways. Investing in and ensuring patient-led diversity, equity and inclusion programs and initiatives focusing on healthcare accessibility, research, and public health initiatives, benefits all with endometriosis, particularly the disabled, BIPOC, LGBTQIA+ within our community. Medical research has been historically white male-dominated in terms of subjects, often excluding trans men, women, particularly Black women and women of color, which is harmful to the endometriosis community. Allocating more funding for research that is not awarded to the same pharmaceutical companies and researchers time and time again is also critical in the quest to come up with a deeper understanding of endometriosis and novel treatments.

3 **Do no harm.** Creating laws that protect access to needed healthcare, particularly necessary reproductive healthcare, including abortion, miscarriage care, and infertility treatments, is crucial for endometriosis patients. Instead of limiting or banning access to care, leaving medical decisions and treatments to endometriosis patients, with the input of their providers, helps protect our community from further medical trauma and harm.

Examples of Goals for Academic Institutional Interventions

1 **Accommodations and flexibility:** Creating an environment where students with endometriosis and other chronic health conditions are met by teachers, administrators and staff with flexibility and not shamed, guilted, or penalized by teachers, administrators and staff, will keep students safe from emotional abuse and gaslighting. Accommodations for endometriosis students can look like close parking, absence, assignment and testing flexibility, and online learning. Students shouldn't be at the mercy of each individual teacher in terms of receiving flexibility. There should be clarity surrounding protective policies and advocates in every school who can help students navigate these challenges.

2 **Education for staff:** At the very least, every school nurse and counselor should be educated on endometriosis and the

emotional and physical impact it has on students. These staff members should be able to help advocate for and support students when they are in need.
3 **Education for students:** Every student should have access to comprehensive health education, including sexual and reproductive health, as well as multidisciplinary physical and mental health resources and education. Endometriosis needs to be a part of this education. This comprehensive health education should also help create a culture of empathy and not only educate students on their own physical and mental health, but how to show empathy for others who are struggling with health issues.

Examples of Goals for Employer Interventions

1 **Physically safe work environment:** Employers can make sure the environments are safe and appropriate when they have the capacity to do so, such as mandating allotted breaks, menstrual products in the bathrooms, work environments with plenty of bathrooms and available offices near bathrooms. They can also offer modifications to the work environment, such as standing desks, special chairs, revised lighting or temperature, to help workers with chronic pain. Flexible work hours can allow workers to have early morning or late afternoon doctors' appointments, while also allowing time to get work completed. Also, work environments free from environmental toxins are incredibly important for everyone, but especially for endometriosis patients.
2 **Emotionally safe work environment:** Employers can respect the dignity and worth of every employee and show their employees empathy by creating a culture where employees regulate their emotions and respect boundaries to promote a healthy work-life balance. The environment must also be inclusive and not discriminate against employees for any reason or punish them for any illness or disability.
3 **Comprehensive benefits:** Employers can offer comprehensive benefits to assist endometriosis patients, such as flexible work

from home policies when possible, comprehensive health insurance benefits that include fertility care and mental healthcare, fair wages, and paid sick leave to name a few.

As individual patients and part of a greater endometriosis patient advocacy community, we need to ask critical questions to explore if our society, government, academic institutions and employers are meeting our needs and keeping us safe from harm. These entities need to work with patient advocates to create interventions to help us thrive.

From Harm to Hope: Fulfilling Our Own Needs

Moving across the country for a new job opportunity was really hard at first. The almost 3,000 miles between me, my family and my childhood friends created a physical boundary and distance that took some time to adjust to. It was also hard to leave my medical team that had helped treat my endometriosis for the past decade.

I moved to California because my new job is a hybrid position, where I could work remotely 75% of the time. It also has better health benefits. I also moved because I started to feel stuck. Despite being very close with my family and friends, there was always some drama that I was expected to fix. No one understood, or even tried to empathize with, all that I have been going through due to my endometriosis. I was constantly asked to be the family therapist, financial advisor, conflict mediator, and caretaker. I was not only expected at every Sunday family dinner, I was obligated to cook and clean for it as well. As the oldest of three siblings, my parents made me feel like their well-being and success was my responsibility, even though they are all adults. My therapist used terms such as co-dependent and enmeshed to describe my family. My family, who has never been to therapy, prefers to use words like close-knit, selfless, and loyal!

These 3,000 miles that now separate us is a natural boundary from the expectations of my family that relieves me from the shame and guilt I used to feel when putting my needs first. Working remotely and not commuting to the middle of New York City every day has also brought me more peace. This job came with a slight pay cut, but I feel like I have gained a better quality of life. I have started to garden and fill my space with plants. My health is still

a struggle, and I am working on building a new multidisciplinary team, but with this new move, I feel more hopeful than I have been in a long time.
  –Gia, age 32

When I was younger, I carried a lot of guilt and pressure to show up in ways that I didn't have the capacity for. I stayed in relationships that demanded more than I had to give. I put a lot of pressure on myself to attend extended family events, even if I was feeling sick or exhausted. The relationships that felt unhealthy eventually ended when I stopped giving. I began to prioritize my time and energy, which meant I had to grieve the loss of working on relationships with those outside of my immediate circle. It has been hard at times feeling judged or dismissed by people who take my absence or perceived neglect personally.

Over the years, I have learned to embrace the misguided persona that people assign to me, especially if it means that I am protecting myself from harm and getting my needs met. In the exam room, I am *that* difficult patient with a degree from Google University who corrects misguided practitioners, asks tough questions, and actively participates in my care. I am the inflexible and aloof family member who sets boundaries with my time and energy when I am not feeling well or am overcapacity. I relish in being the thorny patient advocate who has been told by those in power that maybe if I smile more or make our medical traumas more digestible, our community could get our needs heard and met. I strive to be selfish with my physical and emotional needs. I aspire to take up more space every day. I actively work to care less about what the people who are harming me think of me. I have embodied the cliche that sometimes I have to be the villain in someone else's story to be the hero in my own. I now welcome being labeled difficult. My life and my health depend on it.

Every day in my clinical practice, I see "difficult" endometriosis patients all because they fought to save themselves and keep themselves from physical and emotional harm. They are not difficult people, although what they are going through is incredibly difficult. Their disease is difficult to treat. The medical system they are navigating is difficult. Sometimes their providers are difficult. Their families, their boss, their teachers, their friends can also be difficult.

Life is difficult for them. As we fight to keep ourselves from harm, we are also grieving difficult relationships and systems that are supposed to protect us, yet cause us more harm. We also are grieving our sick bodies, our limited capacities, and the hopes and dreams we once had. It is exhausting. Endometriosis patients are tired.

With so much working against us, it is natural to despair and to lose hope. Hope is a confident and positive feeling or cherished desire regarding the future. For many of us, our future feels bleak and uncertain. When we lose all hope, we can also lose the ability to be resilient, to protect ourselves from harm, to advocate for our needs, and to believe in our inherent self-worth. As people with endometriosis, facing the many challenges this disease brings, our capacity for hope will ebb and flow. The collaborative, multidisciplinary support team we choose to have around us helps us maintain hope, when all hope feels lost.

As a mental health provider in the endometriosis community, I have witnessed empowered patients act as fierce leaders of their support team, as they transition out of despair, enduring less harm and experiencing more hope. When forming a plan on how to create a support team that can meet our many needs, it can be helpful to think about the following questions:

- What are our needs?
    - How can we meet our own needs?
    - What tools and strategies can we use to ensure our needs are met?
- What is our role as captain of our own multidisciplinary team?
    - What are the requirements to be on our support team?
    - Who will be a member of our team and what is their role?

Physiological Needs

- How do we meet our physiological needs?
    - What resources are available that we may not realize?
    - Who or what is keeping us from sleep and rest and how can we better meet these important needs?

Safety Needs

- How do we meet our safety needs?
- How can we improve our health?

- How do we fulfill our educational and vocational needs?
- How do we change relationships with loved ones, providers, or systems that are causing us physical and emotional harm?
  - If we cannot change these harmful relationships, how do we set boundaries with loved ones, providers, or systems that are causing us physical and emotional harm?

Emotional and Social Needs

- How do we meet our emotional and social needs?
  - How can we connect to and find community with others who understand?
- How can we express our emotional and social needs to our loved ones?
- How can we get mental health support?

Self-esteem Needs

- How do we meet our self-esteem needs?
- What gives us value and self-worth?
- How can we feel more independent and more competent?
- How do we preserve our dignity?

Self-actualization Needs

- How do we meet our self-actualization needs?
- What does it mean for us to adapt to our illness?
  - How do we create a life that is sustainable?
- What fixed ideas are holding us back?
  - How can we grieve unhelpful fixed ideas and beliefs so we can be more flexible?
- What brings us despair?
- What are our strengths?
- What boundaries do we need for ourselves to keep us from harm?
- What is our definition of success?
  - What does it mean to be okay?
  - To survive?
  - To thrive?

Our Role as Support Team Leader

Ultimately, we are in charge of our own emotional and physical well-being. Unfortunately, as endometriosis patients, it doesn't always feel this way. We often have needs that feel impossible to meet, many of which feel out of our control. Eradicating endometriosis, changing current endometriosis standards of care, eliminating medical racism and discrimination in the medical industrial complex, putting political leaders in positions of power that can protect the medical autonomy of patients, ensuring expert multidisciplinary healthcare is accessible for all, funding unbiased research, and eliminating poverty are all important needs that contribute to the harm our community faces. While the resolution of these needs aren't in our control, advocates in our community continue to work on these needs as they fight for health equity.

But, we can take steps to improve our lives. Identifying our needs, figuring out which needs we have control over, and setting goals to meet those needs are integral parts of being the leader of our own support team. Feeling empowered to provide guidance, instruction and direction to our support team, while requiring dignity, empathy, respect and influence over the decisions regarding our care will help reduce trauma.

When we have been made to feel powerless, lacking autonomy over our health and well-being, it can feel uncomfortable at first to take back control where we can. But, finding our voice is the first step in having our needs met.

Values Needed to Address Our Needs

Radical Acceptance

Once we grieve and adapt to our reality, we can move towards radical acceptance of that reality. Gaslighting from medical providers, missed diagnosis and mistreatment impact our ability to accept the realities of having endometriosis. A lack of recognition of the challenges of the disease from family members and society in general also interfere with accepting the vast impact of endometriosis. As a result, our inner voice can start to doubt our own lived experience and we gaslight ourselves.

We must develop the ability to ignore those ignorant to our experiences, and believe our own lived experience. Our pain is real. Our fatigue is real. Our disease is real. When we accept that reality we open ourselves up to accept support, set boundaries, and give ourselves grace instead of beating ourselves up and (dys) functioning over our capacity.

Education

As endometriosis patients, we have to become highly educated on our disease and potential comorbidities to keep ourselves safe. We have to read the studies, attend the conferences, and follow the work of patient advocates and expert multidisciplinary medical providers in the endometriosis community. We have to join the online support groups to get more information. This additional mental load that we have to carry is unjust and indicates how the medical industrial complex is failing us. But, education shields us from gaslighting and guides us as leaders of our own support teams.

Self-love

It's so important that we love ourselves the way we would a cherished loved one who was going through a devastating illness. We need to prioritize our own needs, the way we would a loved one's. We need to treat our bodies and minds with kindness and compassion. We need to forgive ourselves for our perceived shortcomings. We need to set aside time for ourselves for joy and relaxation. We need to have empathy for ourselves and our lived experiences. We need to recognize and cherish our good qualities. While the realities of our health and limited physical capacity can be devastating, finding ways to make our love of self unconditional, will help us continue to get our needs met, even at our most hopeless of times.

Advocacy

The gaslighting, emotional abuse, and systemic challenges to getting an endometriosis diagnosis and effective treatments can make us feel voiceless. Yet, time and time again, we are put in positions where our emotional and physical well-being relies on our capacity to advocate for ourselves and our needs. Whether it's asking for a better pain protocol for a medical procedure from our provider, or insisting that we cannot make it to a family event, we are often tasked with having uncomfortable conversations to preserve our health. This can feel especially difficult if we are tired and feeling powerless.

When my patients are anxious about advocating for themselves, I ask them to identify a person, real or fictional, who is a fierce and unapologetic advocate. So far, I've heard examples ranging anywhere from Michelle Obama, to Ruth Bader Ginsburg, to RuPaul and others. We then come up with their own version of that person that they can invoke during their difficult appointment or conversation. We sometimes can more easily be a fierce and unapologetic advocate for the needs of others, but still feel uncomfortable speaking up for our own needs when the time comes. We need to feel empowered to advocate like our physical and emotional well-being depends on it, as it often does.

Peer Support

We cannot do this disease alone. So many of my endometriosis patients come into my office feeling completely hopeless and isolated because there is no one around them, from medical providers to family members, who understand what they are going through. I am often the first person they have met that also has endometriosis.

Connecting with other people who understand what we have gone through helps us feel validated and shields us from gaslighting. Joining an online education or support group, or finding patient advocates on social media can make a positive impact on our well-being. As leaders of our own support team, it is also important to connect with other leaders to hear what has been helpful for them and what has not been helpful. Because endometriosis excision surgery has not been deemed a gynecological subspecialty and current accepted standards of care are outdated, connecting with other patients online can provide insights on who we should recruit for our support team, protecting us from potential emotional and physical harm.

Recruitment

Ideally, as endometriosis patients navigating health challenges, we should be empowered to decide who is worthy enough to be on our support team. Members on our support team must respect our role as team leader, let us make our own decisions, adhere to our boundaries and standards, while showing self-awareness, accountability, empathy and compassion, all essential ingredients for a successful team. Members on our support team must respect our authority to provide guidance, instruction and direction as we look to avoid unnecessary harm.

While it is good to have high standards for our support team members, it is important to note that some of them will fall short. In assessing our own needs, we have to know the ways our team members are meeting our needs or neglecting our needs. We may have a primary care provider who knows nothing about endometriosis, but they are trauma-informed, open to care suggestions, responsive to referrals, needed blood work and imaging. We may have an expert excision surgeon who is not trauma-informed, but is the only provider with his expertise remotely close geographically and is in-network with insurance. This surgeon may meet our physical needs, but increases medical trauma due to poor bedside manner. Our parents may have the capacity to aid us financially, but with that may come a cost that includes emotional abuse, shame, guilt and gaslighting.

When recruiting our support team, we don't always have the clearest choices as we try to balance our physical, emotional, and financial needs. Ultimately, when potential team members fall short, we have to assess if the dynamic of the relationship can change, and if not, if the relationship is ultimately benefiting us more than it is harming us. We have to remember not to internalize any abuse and know when to set up boundaries to keep ourselves safe.

Reframing

Due to gaslighting and abuse, we often have a negative, critical bully inside of us that says mean things to us throughout the day, things that we would never say to other people. Part of meeting our own emotional needs and feeling hopeful is challenging that voice and reframing the harmful things that have been told to us over the years, that we now tell ourselves.

This looks like accepting that taking care of our own needs first is not selfish behavior, but self-preserving behavior, protecting ourselves from harm. This looks like feeling grateful for the healthy support from others rather than feeling guilty or bad about it. This looks like believing that we are not bad or difficult people, but that endometriosis is an incredibly difficult disease. When we tell ourselves we are incompetent or lazy, maybe we can instead assure ourselves we are just tired, overcapacity, and due to being human, imperfect.

Self-awareness

Before we know where to set boundaries, we have to be aware of our feelings and needs. When we are forced to endure abusive and traumatic experiences and environments over time, we often learn to disassociate from our emotional and physical needs and experiences to survive. We start to ignore that inner voice that tells us something is wrong because we learned that expressing those thoughts doesn't change anything, and sometimes makes things worse. When those in power tell us our thoughts, opinions, feelings, lived experiences, don't matter or aren't accurate, we start doubting ourselves and silence our self-awareness.

It's important to reconnect with our self-awareness to understand what is causing us emotional and physical harm, and draining our precious energy and resources. Ultimately, our self-awareness will guide us to setting boundaries.

Boundaries

When we think about what precious resources belong to us that we desperately need boundaries on to protect, we think of:

- our time
- our energy
- our finances
- our emotional and physical health and well-being.

While it may make us feel uncomfortable, setting uncompromising boundaries with those who hurt us, invalidate us, drain us, or make us feel small is an important act of self-preservation. When we become self-aware, we can feel if something is causing us resentment, harming us, or pushing us overcapacity. Coming up with a list of non-negotiables that we will never do again in the name of fiercely protecting our physical and mental health can give us freedom from the things that are oppressing us. Feeling empowered to fire medical providers who no longer serve our best interests, or worse, harm us, can feel empowering. Putting up strict boundaries with family members, friends, or coworkers who cause us harm or drain our energy can help us reclaim our scarce resources.

Flexibility

Our society often makes us feel like we have to be self-sacrificing, super-productive, overworked and overscheduled to hold value. Our family culture can reflect those values as well, and sometimes even place our value on how much we give of ourselves to our family. Growing up, it is natural to be influenced by the ideas we marinate in, as we try to understand what defines us and what gives us value. When we are impacted by endometriosis and cannot finish law school, have children, give expected time and energy to family members, keep up with a rigorous job, or get married, we start to believe that we don't have value, due to the narrow definition of value we have always been given. If we believe we no longer have value, we feel hopeless and meeting our needs can feel pointless.

We first need to give ourselves the space to properly grieve. Grieving what we have always wanted, dreamed of and cannot have is an integral part of adapting to endometriosis. Grieving and processing the losses we experience can take time, and those feelings of sadness may reappear as we go through life. But, when our value is tied to us achieving things we don't have the capacity for, we not only have to grieve our losses, but we have to rebuild the foundation of who we are outside of society's and our family's expectations of us. This is a painful process, but at the end of it, we get to define what gives us value. We get to decide what it means to thrive. When we give ourselves the grace of flexibility to adapt our goals to our current capacity, and recognize our inherent value, we can feel more hopeful, and less stuck.

It takes a lot of energy, courage and resilience to be the leader of our own support team. There are going to be times when our grief, anger, depression and anxiety feel all-consuming. We are going to feel pressured to do things we do not have the capacity for, and also, will need things from our body we are not capable of. We may feel disillusioned as we expend an exuberant amount of resources that we don't have, with the hope and promise of achieving wellness, only for it to not help, or even cause more harm. Even with the best care, which is inaccessible for many, endometriosis and the comorbidities that come with it are challenging and scary. Our ability to let go of self-blame, and adapt to what is within and out of our control, will help us integrate all aspects of the disease into our lives and adapt to our ever changing reality. As endometriosis patients, keeping ourselves from emotional and physical harm, while maintaining hope, is a lifelong pursuit.

As a social worker and patient advocate, what has touched me the most is our community's continued capacity for hope and resilience through the many challenges this disease brings. I see hope as a commitment to ourselves to try to make things better, not only for ourselves, but for those in our community coming after us. As patients, we hope every day in very big and small ways.

Patient advocates whose bodies are tired and aching, wake up every day and continue to try to roll the big boulder up the advocacy hill, making progress on education, research, systemic support, and awareness, while also being subjected to criticism and invalidation. They continue because they hope that their efforts will keep others from the trauma and harm they have experienced.

We exert hope in small ways when we get out of bed, eat a meal or take a shower. Hope is expressed through seeing a new medical provider, overcoming anxiety, trying new things, and letting go of things that do not serve us anymore and are weighing us down, like a toxic job or relationship. Hope helps us believe in ourselves and recognize our strengths.

Endometriosis has taken many things from me throughout my life. It's a disease that ravages a person, decimating our organs, fertility, and quality of life. What brings me hope is thinking about what endometriosis cannot take away from me or others in our community. Despite all it has robbed from us, we still have value. Despite our limited capacities, we still have strengths. We are worthy of love, dignity, and joy because we exist. Maybe the greatest boundary of all that we need to set is with the disease itself. We may not have complete control over what the disease takes from us, but through support, self-love, and self-care we can make sure it doesn't ravage every bit of us.

Appendix A
Endometriosis Treatment and Support Protocol for all Providers

At every single endometriosis conference I have been to in the past decade, there are inevitably endometriosis excision surgeons debating over whether utilizing the robot during laparoscopic excision surgery is superior to not using the robot. Fertility specialists often argue whether endometriosis excision surgery is needed to improve fertility, or if patients should go straight to IVF. Mental health providers may disagree on whether or not Cognitive Behavioral Therapy is more useful than Eye Movement Desensitization Reprocessing Therapy (EMDR) to help patients with medical trauma. While these debates can be constructive and help us understand how providers approach the challenges we face as patients, it often feels like these arguments detract from tackling the universal harms in approaches to care.

Providers have different tools to offer endometriosis patients as we navigate the medical system to address our needs related to endometriosis. Providers who are mentally healthy are flexible, collaborative, and put the needs of the patient ahead of their own. Whether an emergency medicine physician, a gastroenterologist, a pelvic floor therapist, a surgeon, a fertility specialist, or a mental health provider, there are universal approaches to care when helping endometriosis patients fulfill their needs to reduce harm.

1 **Validation:** Every single healthcare provider, from a primary care provider to the most knowledgeable endometriosis excision surgeon, has the ability to provide some healing to patients by simply showing that they hear where we are coming from and believe our lived experience. By giving us space to talk about our pain, believing what we say, and then verbally acknowledging it, our medical trauma is reduced.
2 **Education:** After our pain and symptoms are acknowledged and validated, educating us on what endometriosis is and all of its

potential implications is incredibly affirming and helps us begin to process and adapt to what may be going on in our bodies. To educate the millions of patients with this disease, providers have to first educate themselves. Because endometriosis is a multisystemic disease, any healthcare provider who treats those assigned female at birth needs to be familiar with the disease and its implications for their practice. Gastroenterologists need to be able to recognize potential bowel endometriosis and educate patients on the disease and implications. Urologists need to be able to suspect endometriosis on the bladder and ureters. Individual providers need to recognize the misinformation and the gaps in education they have received that have caused harm to their patients. Education surrounding endometriosis needs to come from patient advocates and expert multidisciplinary providers in the community. The more providers know, the more patients are educated and empowered.

3 **Connection:** As a social worker in the field, and a patient myself, I have witnessed first-hand the isolation endometriosis patients face and the hope that can come from connecting to other patients and nonprofits in the community. This is especially important for Black, Indigenous, People of Color, as well as patients who are a part of the LGBTQIA+ community. Healthcare offices are filled with pamphlets explaining various diseases, vaccinations, and medical treatments from pharmaceutical companies. Endometriosis pamphlets made by patient advocates and expert multidisciplinary providers, offering basic disease information and local and national patient support resources would help patients feel more connected and less isolated.

4 **Intervention:** By definition, intervention means to improve a situation. The interventions that healthcare providers offer for endometriosis patients must be trauma-informed to not make the situation worse. To truly improve a situation for endometriosis patients, providers must first have accurate information surrounding endometriosis. Providers must listen to our presenting challenges, as well as our overall goals. Providers must then supply true informed consent, which means giving

patients thorough information regarding our suspected or confirmed endometriosis, providing their strengths and limitations as the treating provider, risks and benefits of the treatments they can offer, as well as what other providers with different skills can offer. Not intervening, and referring a patient to a more experienced provider who has more tools to help a patient reach their goals is a form of intervention that can improve the situation.

5 **Specialization/collaboration:** As a mental health provider to endometriosis patients, I feel confident that I single-handedly cannot meet all of the emotional, social, and physical needs of all of my patients. In my practice, that sometimes looks like referring a patient to another therapist that can offer EMDR for medical trauma or a psychiatrist that can prescribe medications to help support mental health. If I have a patient already in long-term therapy for an eating disorder or substance use disorder, I work with my patient and their primary therapist on interventions that do not impinge on other mental health goals, as we work to navigate endometriosis. Every provider has the opportunity to critically reflect with each patient on their goals and needs, and then provide referrals for and collaborate with other healthcare providers who can best meet those needs. Multidisciplinary care and provider collaboration reduces medical trauma for patients with chronic pain and chronic illness.

6 **Advocacy:** Providers who are reading this book now have the knowledge to prevent harm and provide better care for endometriosis patients. Providers can work with their patients to be excellent advocates for their care. I have had to call other mental health providers and educate them on endometriosis after they have dismissed or invalidated a patient's lived experience due to their ignorance surrounding the disease. Many expert endometriosis excision surgeons talk about the harm they have seen when operating on patients who have had surgery done by an unskilled provider. Some but not all of these surgeons have confronted the less skilled providers on the harm they caused.

The American Medical Association's Ethics Code explicitly states that all physicians have an ethical obligation to report colleagues who they suspect are harming patients.

- What can providers do to make sure their colleagues aren't harming endometriosis patients?
- What can providers do to make sure the practices they work in aren't harming endometriosis patients?
- What can providers do to make sure the medical organizations they pay dues to aren't harming endometriosis patients?

Healthcare providers and the medical industrial complex they work within have the capacity to reduce harm for and instill hope in endometriosis patients and meet their needs. Providers have the opportunity to demand unbiased, patient-led, expert informed multidisciplinary endometriosis education from the medical organizations that approve standards of care and continuing education credits. The first step to doing no harm is recognizing that harm is being done and working with those of us who have been harmed on creating better care.

Acknowledgments

There are so many people I need to thank who have helped make this book possible. I would like to first thank my family and friends, especially Billy and Annie, not only for their support and encouragement throughout the writing process, but for the empathy and validation they have shown me over the years as a person navigating multiple chronic illnesses. Thank you for making me feel loved.

A special thank you to my cheerleaders at Inner Solutions Counseling who have believed in me and made my transition into a full-time mental health provider and author a celebration. Thank you to nutritionist Riley Burns, MS, RDN, LDN for her insights into eating disorders.

A special thank you to Rachel Landes and Sheldon Press for making my dream of writing a book focused on endometriosis and mental health come true. You have helped make an invisible disease more visible. I am so appreciative of your fierce commitment to the wellness of our community through publishing this book.

Although I have been doing this work for the past 15 years, there are patient advocates who I allude to in this book that started this work long before I even knew what endometriosis was. A heartfelt thank you to my mentor and friend, Heather Guidone BCPA, whose exhaustive work continues to pave the path that subsequent advocates in this community walk. To other patient advocates and multidisciplinary providers I have been in community with, fighting for change, I am grateful for your tireless dedication, inspiration, and camaraderie.

While the patient narratives in this book aren't from actual patients, they could be. The stories written are universal, assembled from pieces of loss, medical trauma, invalidation, and harm that have been recurrent themes in the lives of my patients and those throughout the community. My patients show up for sessions hoping they will not be harmed, even though they have been harmed time and time again by a multitude of providers over the years. It is an honor to be a clinical social worker in the endometriosis, infertility, pregnancy loss, and chronic illness communities.

In a heartbeat, I would trade this book for a cure. My greatest hope is that one day this book will be obsolete and we can prevent all harm before it begins. Until then, I am grateful for all of the patients, loved ones, and providers who are reading this publication. Let us keep empathetically collaborating to reduce harm for all those who are suffering.

Resources

A complete and updated list of resources can be found on www.CaseyBerna.com

Patient Resources Mentioned In the Book

Endo Black
https://www.endoblack.org
Project Endo
https://www.projectendo.org
MISE Program
https://miseireland.ie/
EndoRISE
https://ctendorise.org
Rape, Abuse & Incest National Network
https://rainn.org/resources
PCOS Challenge: The National Polycystic Ovary Syndrome Association
https://pcoschallenge.org
The Menopause Society
https://menopause.org
The Autoimmune Association
https://autoimmune.org
Suicide and Crisis Lifeline
https://988lifeline.org
Suicide Prevention UK
https://spuk.org.uk/national-suicide-prevention-helpline/
The Trevor Project
https://www.thetrevorproject.org
The International Association for Premenstrual Disorders
https://iapmd.org
National Eating Disorders Association
https://www.nationaleatingdisorders.org

Other Patient-Driven Nonprofits and Resources

Gynoqueer
https://endoqueer.com
Extra Pelvic Not Rare
https://extrapelvicnotrare.org
The Endometriosis Coalition
https://www.theendo.co
Lela Foundation
https://www.lelafoundation.org
Latinas Con Endo
https://www.instagram.com/latinasconendo/
Sister Girl Foundation
https://www.sister-girl.org
The Endometriosis Research Center
https://www.endocenter.org
Barbados Association Of Endometriosis and P.C.O.S.
https://endoandpcosbb.com
The Endometriosis Association of Ireland
https://www.endometriosis.ie
The Endometriosis Summit
https://theendometriosissummit.com
The Endo Girls Blog
https://endogirlblog.com
Nancy's Nook Facebook Education Group
https://www.facebook.com/groups/418136991574617
American End to Endo Project
https://endofendoproject.org/
The Childless Collective
https://childlesscollective.com
AllPaths Family Building
https://allpathsfb.org/new-name-same-mission/
RESOLVE
https://resolve.org
Recurrent Pregnancy Loss Association
https://rplassociation.org/
The White Dress Project
https://www.thewhitedressproject.org/

Interstitial Cystitis Association
https://www.ichelp.org/
Postpartum Support International
https://postpartum.net/
Dysautonomia International
https://www.dysautonomiainternational.org
The Ehler-Danlos Society
https://www.ehlers-danlos.com/
POTS UK
https://www.potsuk.org/about-pots/diagnosis/

Supporting Research

Chapter 1: Endometriosis, Symptoms, Treatments and Diagnosis

Guidone HC. Collaboration is key in managing endometriosis. BMJ 2025; 388:q2725 doi:10.1136/bmj.q2725

Fryer J, Mason-Jones AJ, Woodward A. Understanding diagnostic delay for endometriosis: A scoping review. medRxiv 2024.01.08.24300988; doi:https://doi.org/10.1101/2024.01.08.24300988

International Working Group of AAGL, ESGE, ESHRE and WES; Tomassetti C, Johnson NP, Petrozza J, Abrao MS, Einarsson JI, Horne AW, Lee TTM, Missmer S, Vermeulen N, Zondervan KT, Grimbizis G, De Wilde RL. An international terminology for endometriosis, 2021. Hum Reprod Open. 2021 Oct 22; 2021(4):hoab029. doi: 10.1093/hropen/hoab029. PMID: 34693033; PMCID: PMC8530702.

Bao C, Wang H, Fang H. Genomic evidence supports the recognition of endometriosis as an inflammatory systemic disease and reveals disease-specific therapeutic potentials of targeting neutrophil degranulation. Front Immunol. 2022 Mar 23;13:758440. doi: 10.3389/fimmu.2022.758440. PMID: 35401535; PMCID: PMC8983833.

Troncon JK, Zani AC, Vieira AD, Poli-Neto OB, Nogueira AA, Rosa-E-Silva JC. Endometriosis in a patient with mayer-rokitansky-küster-hauser syndrome. Case Rep Obstet Gynecol. 2014; 2014:376231. doi: 10.1155/2014/376231. Epub 2014 Dec 30. PMID: 25610677; PMCID: PMC4293785.

Pickett C, Foster WG, Agarwal S. Current endometriosis care and opportunities for improvement. Reprod Fertil. 2023 Jul 1;4(3):e220091. doi: 10.1530/RAF-22-0091. Epub ahead of print. PMID: 37402150; PMCID: PMC10448566.

Cano-Herrera G, Salmun Nehmad S, Ruiz de Chávez Gascón J, Méndez Vionet A, van Tienhoven XA, Osorio Martínez MF, Muleiro Alvarez M, Vasco Rivero MX, López Torres MF, Barroso Valverde MJ, Noemi Torres I, Cruz Olascoaga A, Bautista Gonzalez MF, Sarkis Nehme JA, Vélez Rodríguez I, Murguiondo Pérez R, Salazar FE, Sierra Bronzon AG, Rivera Rosas EG, ... Cabrera Carranco R. Endometriosis: A comprehensive analysis of the pathophysiology, treatment, and nutritional aspects, and its repercussions on the quality of life of patients. Biomedicines. 2024 12;7:1476. https://doi.org/10.3390/biomedicines12071476

Imperiale L, Nisolle M, Noël JC, Fastrez M. Three types of endometriosis: Pathogenesis, diagnosis and treatment. State of the art. J Clin Med.

2023 Jan 28;12(3):994. doi: 10.3390/jcm12030994. PMID: 36769642; PMCID: PMC9918005.

Chauhan S, More A, Chauhan V, Kathane A. Endometriosis: A review of clinical diagnosis, treatment, and pathogenesis. Cureus. 2022;Sep 6; 14(9):e28864. doi: 10.7759/cureus.28864. PMID: 36225394; PMCID: PMC9537113.

Bontempo AC, Schiff GD. Diagnosing diagnostic error of endometriosis: A secondary analysis of patient experiences from a mixed-methods survey. BMJ Open Quality 2025;14:e003121.

Chapron C, Pietin-Vialle C, Borghese B, Davy C, Foulot H, Chopin N. Associated ovarian endometrioma is a marker for greater severity of deeply infiltrating endometriosis. Fertility and sterility, 2009;92;2;453–457, ISSN 0015-0282, https://doi.org/10.1016/j.fertnstert.2008.06.003.

Andres MP, Arcoverde FVL, Souza CCC, Fernandes LFC, Abrão MS, Kho RM. Extrapelvic endometriosis: A systematic review. J Minim Invasive Gynecol. 2020 Feb;27(2):373–389. doi: 10.1016/j.jmig.2019.10.004. Epub 2019 Oct 13. PMID: 31618674.

Allaire C, Bedaiwy MA, Yong PJ. Diagnosis and management of endometriosis. CMAJ. 2023 Mar 14;195(10):E363-E371. doi: 10.1503/cmaj. 220637. PMID: 36918177; PMCID: PMC10120420.

Secosan C, Balulescu L, Brasoveanu S, Balint O, Pirtea P, Dorin G, Pirtea L. Endometriosis in menopause-renewed attention on a controversial disease. Diagnostics (Basel). 2020 Feb 29;10(3):134. doi: 10.3390/diagnostics10030134. PMID: 32121424; PMCID: PMC7151055.

Rizk B, Fischer AS, Lotfy HA, Turki R, Zahed HA, Malik R, Holliday CP, Glass A, Fishel H, Soliman MY, Herrera D. Recurrence of endometriosis after hysterectomy. Facts Views Vis Obgyn. 2014;6(4):219–227. PMID: 25593697; PMCID: PMC4286861.

Vallée A, Ceccaldi PF, Carbonnel M, Feki A, Ayoubi JM. Pollution and endometriosis: A deep dive into the environmental impacts on women's health. BJOG. 2024 Mar;131(4):401–414. doi: 10.1111/1471-0528.17687. Epub 2023 Oct 9. PMID: 37814514.

Signorile PG, Baldi F, Bussani R, Viceconte R, Bulzomi P, D'Armiento M, D'Avino A, Baldi A. Embryologic origin of endometriosis: Analysis of 101 human female fetuses. J Cell Physiol. 2012 Apr;227(4):1653–6. doi: 10.1002/jcp.22888. PMID: 21678420.

Takada L, Kawano T, Yano K, Iwamoto Y, Ogata M, Kedoin C, Murakami M, Sugita K, Onishi S, Muto M, Kirishima M, Tanimoto A, Ieiri S. Ovarian endometrioma: A report of a pediatric case diagnosed prior to menstruation. Surg Case Rep. 2024 Jun 20;10(1):152. doi: 10.1186/s40792-024-01951-5. PMID: 38898208; PMCID: PMC11187045.

Brosens I, Gordts S, Benagiano G. Endometriosis in adolescents is a hidden, progressive and severe disease that deserves attention, not just compassion. Hum Reprod. 2013 Aug;28(8):2026–31. doi: 10.1093/humrep/det243. Epub 2013 Jun 5. PMID: 23739215; PMCID: PMC3712662.

Dysmenorrhea and endometriosis in the adolescent. ACOG Committee Opinion No. 760. American College of Obstetricians and Gynecologists. Obstet Gynecol 2018;132:e249–58.

Requadt E, Nahlik AJ, Jacobsen A, Ross WT. Patient experiences of endometriosis diagnosis: A mixed methods approach. BJOG: An International Journal of Obstetrics & Gynaecology 2024;131(7);941–951.

Chapter 2: Why is Endometriosis Uniquely Challenging to Treat?

Langmann E, Kainradl AC, Weßel M, Rokvity A. Endometriosis in later life: An intersectional analysis from the perspective of epistemic injustice. Med Healthcare Philos. 2025 Mar;28(1):151–159. doi: 10.1007/s11019-024-10245-4. Epub 2024 Dec 20. PMID: 39704896; PMCID: PMC11805771.

Coxon L, Demetriou L, Vincent K. Current developments in endometriosis-associated pain. Cell Rep Med. 2024 Oct 15;5(10):101769. doi: 10.1016/j.xcrm.2024.101769. PMID: 39413731; PMCID: PMC11513828.

Duncan J-M, Delara R, Ranieri G, Wasson M. Management of endometriosis: A call to multidisciplinary approach. Journal of Osteopathic Medicine 2024. https://doi.org/10.1515/jom-2024-0105.

Wójcik M, Szczepaniak R, Placek K. Physiotherapy management in endometriosis. Int J Environ Res Public Health. 2022 Dec 2;19(23):16148. doi: 10.3390/ijerph192316148. PMID: 36498220; PMCID: PMC9740037.

Price and Prejudice: Reimbursement of Surgical Care on Male Versus Female Anatomies.

Penn M, Colley D, P Koirala P, King L, Fitzgerald J. Journal of Women's Health. 2025 Feb;34(12).

Mandeville J, Pollack AZ, Kornegay L, Gupta J. Stigma and discrimination experienced by Black women with endometriosis in the Washington, DC, Metropolitan area: A pilot of the ENDO-served study. Int J Gynaecol Obstet. 2025 Mar 1. doi: 10.1002/ijgo.70042. Epub ahead of print. PMID: 40022574.

Amutah C, Greenidge K, Mante A, Munyikwa M, Surya SL, Higginbotham E, Jones DS, Lavizzo-Mourey R, Roberts D, Tsai J. Misrepresenting race—the role of medical schools in propagating physician bias. N Engl J Med. 2021;384(9):872–878. doi:10.1056/NEJMms2025768.

Kashyap A, Aziz M, Sun TY et al. Investigating racial disparities in drug prescriptions for patients with endometriosis. npj Womens Health 3, 6 (2025). https://doi.org/10.1038/s44294-025-00053-3.

Bougie O, Healey J, Singh SS. Behind the times: revisiting endometriosis and race. Am J Obstet Gynecol. 2019 Jul;221(1):35.e1-35.e5. doi: 10.1016/j.ajog.2019.01.238. Epub 2019 Feb 6. PMID: 30738028.

Weiss MS, Marsh EE. Navigating Unequal Paths: Racial Disparities in the Infertility Journey. Obstet Gynecol. 2023 Oct 1;142(4):940–947. doi: 10.1097/AOG.0000000000005354. PMID: 37678890; PMCID: PMC10510808.

Alexander AL, Strohl AE, Rieder S, Holl J, Barber EL. Examining Disparities in Route of Surgery and Postoperative Complications in Black Race and Hysterectomy. Obstet Gynecol. 2019 Jan;133(1):6–12. doi: 10.1097/AOG.0000000000002990. PMID: 30531569; PMCID: PMC6326082.

Casanova-Perez R, Apodaca C, Bascom E, Mohanraj D, Lane C, Vidyarthi D, Beneteau E, Sabin J, Pratt W, Weibel N, Hartzler AL. Broken down by bias: Healthcare biases experienced by BIPOC and LGBTQ+ patients. AMIA Annu Symp Proc. 2022 Feb 21;2021:275–284. PMID: 35308990; PMCID: PMC8861755.

Eder C, Roomaney R. Transgender and non-binary people's experience of endometriosis. J Health Psychol. 2024 Aug 10:13591053241266249. doi: 10.1177/13591053241266249. Epub ahead of print. PMID: 39127882.

Chapter 3: Endometriosis: Sexual and Reproductive Health

Kendell RE. Hysteria, Editor(s): Smelser NJ, Baltes PB. International encyclopedia of the social & behavioral sciences. Pergamon, 2001, 7133–7138, ISBN 9780080430768, https://doi.org/10.1016/B0-08-043076-7/03725-6.

Mohd Tohit NF, Haque M. Forbidden conversations: A comprehensive exploration of taboos in sexual and reproductive health. Cureus. 2024 Aug 12;16(8):e66723. doi: 10.7759/cureus.66723. PMID: 39139803; PMCID: PMC11319820.

Pluchino N, Wenger J-M, Petignat P, Tal R, Bolmont M, Taylor HS, Bianchi-Demicheli F. Sexual function in endometriosis patients and their partners: Effect of the disease and consequences of treatment. Human Reproduction Update, 22;6(20) Nov 2016;762–774.

Zussman L, Zussman S, Sunley R, Bjornson E. Sexual response after hysterectomy-oophorectomy: Recent studies and reconsideration of psychogenesis. American Journal of Obstetrics and Gynecology, 1981;140;7;725–729, ISSN 0002-9378, https://doi.org/10.1016/0002-9378(81)90730-4.

Practice Committee of the American Society for Reproductive Medicine. Definition of infertility: a committee opinion. Fertility and Sterility, 2023;120(6);1170.

Practice Committee of the American Society for Reproductive Medicine. Endometriosis and infertility: A committee opinion. Fertility and sterility, 2012;98(3);591–598.

Nezhat C, Khoyloo F, Tsuei A, Armani E, Page B, Rduch T, Nezhat C. The prevalence of endometriosis in patients with unexplained infertility. J Clin Med. 2024 Jan 13;13(2):444. doi: 10.3390/jcm13020444. PMID: 38256580; PMCID: PMC11326441.

Kirubarajan A, Patel P, Leung S, Park B, Sierra S. Cultural competence in fertility care for lesbian, gay, bisexual, transgender, and queer people: A systematic review of patient and provider perspectives. Fertility and Sterility, 2021;115;5;1294–1301, ISSN 0015-0282, https://doi.org/10.1016/j.fertnstert.2020.12.002.

Gollapudi M, Thomas A, Yogarajah A, Ospina D, Daher JC, Rahman A, Santistevan L, Patel RV, Abraham J, Oommen SG, Siddiqui HF. Understanding the interplay between premenstrual dysphoric disorder (PMDD) and female sexual dysfunction (FSD). Cureus. 2024 Jun 20; 16(6):e62788. doi: 10.7759/cureus.62788. PMID: 39036127; PMCID: PMC11260262.

Boje AD, Egerup P, Westergaard D, Bertelsen MMF, Nyegaard M, Hartwell D, Lidegaard Ø, Nielsen HS. Endometriosis is associated with pregnancy loss: A nationwide historical cohort study. Fertil Steril. 2023 May;119(5):826835. doi: 10.1016/j.fertnstert.2022.12.042. Epub 2023 Jan 3. PMID: 36608920.

Palomba S, Santagni S, Gibbins K, Battista La Sala G, Silver RM. Reproductive BioMedicine Online, 2016 33;5;612–628.

Mukherjee, S, Velez E, Baird, DD, Savitz DA, Hartmann KE. Risk of miscarriage among black women and white women in a US prospective cohort study. American Journal of Epidemiology. 2013;177(11);1271–1278.

Farren J, Jalmbrant M, Falconieri N, Mitchell-Jones N, Bobdiwala S, Al-Memar M, Tapp S, Van Calster B, Wynants L, Timmerman D, Bourne T. Posttraumatic stress, anxiety and depression following miscarriage and ectopic pregnancy: a multicenter, prospective, cohort study. Am J Obstet Gynecol. 2020 Apr;222(4):367.e1-367.e22. doi: 10.1016/j.ajog.2019.10.102. Epub 2019 Dec 13. PMID: 31953115.

Singh M, Wambua S, Lee SI, Okoth K, Wang Z, Fazla F, Fayaz A, Eastwood KA, Nelson-Piercy C, Nirantharakumar K, Crowe F; MuM-PreDiCT. Autoimmune diseases and adverse pregnancy outcomes: An umbrella review. Lancet. 2023 Nov;402 Suppl 1:S84. doi: 10.1016/S0140-6736(23)02128-1. PMID: 37997130.

Breintoft K, Arendt LH, Uldbjerg N, Glavind MT, Forman A, Henriksen TB. Endometriosis and preterm birth: A Danish cohort study. Acta Obstet Gynecol Scand. 2022 Apr;101(4):417–423. doi: 10.1111/aogs.14336. Epub 2022 Feb 26. PMID: 35218204; PMCID: PMC9564798.

Piriyev E, Römer T. Coincidence of uterine malformations and endometriosis: A clinically relevant problem? Arch Gynecol Obstet. 2020 Nov;302(5):1237–1241. doi: 10.1007/s00404-020-05750-9. Epub 2020 Aug 20. PMID: 32816056.

Breintoft K, Pinnerup R, Henriksen TB, Rytter D, Uldbjerg N, Forman A, Arendt LH. Endometriosis and risk of adverse pregnancy outcome: A systematic review and meta-analysis. J Clin Med. 2021 Feb 9;10(4):667. doi: 10.3390/jcm10040667. PMID: 33572322; PMCID: PMC7916165.

Howell EA. Reducing disparities in severe maternal morbidity and mortality. Clin Obstet Gynecol. 2018 Jun;61(2):387–399. doi: 10.1097/GRF.0000000000000349. PMID: 29346121; PMCID: PMC5915910.

Blom EA, Jansen PW, Verhulst FC, Hofman A, Raat H, Jaddoe VW, Coolman M, Steegers EA, Tiemeier H. Perinatal complications increase the risk of postpartum depression. The Generation R Study. BJOG. 2010 Oct;117(11):1390–1398. doi: 10.1111/j.1471-0528.2010.02660.x. PMID: 20682022.

Tahirkheli NN, Cherry AS, Tackett AP, McCaffree MA, Gillaspy SR. Postpartum depression on the neonatal intensive care unit: Current perspectives. Int J Womens Health. 2014 Nov 24;6:975–987. doi: 10.2147/IJWH.S54666. PMID: 25473317; PMCID: PMC4247145.

Simpkins JW, Brown K, Bae S, Ratka A. Role of ethnicity in the expression of features of hot flashes. Maturitas. 2009 Aug 20;63(4):341–346. doi: 10.1016/j.maturitas.2009.06.002. Epub 2009 Jul 9. PMID: 19592184; PMCID: PMC7050441.

Havers-Borgersen E, Hartwell D, Butt JH, Oestergaard L, Koeber LV, Fosboel EL. Endometriosis, a prevalent disease, is associated with significant cardiac disease. European Heart Journal 2024 Oct 45;Supplement_1, ehae666.3074.

Ding DC, Tsai IJ, Hsu CY, Wang JH, Lin SZ. Hysterectomy is associated with higher risk of coronary artery disease: A nationwide retrospective cohort study in Taiwan. Medicine (Baltimore). 2018 Apr;97(16):e0421. doi: 10.1097/MD.0000000000010421. PMID: 29668602; PMCID: PMC5916687.

Yuk J, Kim BG, Lee BK, Seo J, Kim GS, Min K, Lee HY, Byun YS, Kim BO, Seung-Woo Yang S-W, Kim M-H, Yoon S-H, Seo Y-S. Association of early hysterectomy with risk of cardiovascular disease in Korean women. JAMA Netw Open. 2023;6(6):e2317145. doi:10.1001/jamanetworkopen.2023.17145.

Parsa S, Noroozpoor R, Dehghanbanadaki H, Khateri S, Moradi Y. Endometriosis and risk of cardiovascular disease: A systematic review and meta-analysis. BMC Public Health 2025;25;245. https://doi.org/10.1186/s12889-025-21486-0.

Chapter 4: It's Almost Never Just Endo: Common Comorbidities

Kunz G, Beil D, Huppert P, Noe M, Kissler S, Leyendecker G. Adenomyosis in endometriosis—prevalence and impact on fertility. Evidence from magnetic resonance imaging. Hum Reprod. 2005 Aug;20(8):2309–2316. doi: 10.1093/humrep/dei021. Epub 2005 May 26. PMID: 15919780.

Uimari O, Nazri H, Tapmeier T. Endometriosis and uterine fibroids (Leiomyomata): Comorbidity, risks and implications. Front Reprod Health. 2021 Oct 26;3:750018. doi: 10.3389/frph.2021.750018. PMID: 36304022; PMCID: PMC9580755.

Butrick CW. Patients with chronic pelvic pain: Endometriosis or interstitial cystitis/painful bladder syndrome? JSLS. 2007 Apr–Jun;11(2):182–9. PMID: 17761077; PMCID: PMC3015726.

Schliep KC, Ghabayen L, Shaaban M, Hughes FR, Pollack AZ, Stanford JB, Brady KA, Kiser A, Peterson CM. Examining the co-occurrence of endometriosis and polycystic ovarian syndrome. AJOG Glob Rep. 2023 Aug 28;3(3):100259. doi: 10.1016/j.xagr.2023.100259. PMID: 37663310; PMCID: PMC10472311.

Boneva RS, Lin JS, Wieser F, Nater UM, Ditzen B, Taylor RN, Unger ER. Endometriosis as a comorbid condition in chronic fatigue syndrome (CFS): Secondary analysis of data from a CFS case-control Study. Front Pediatr. 2019 May 21;7:195. doi: 10.3389/fped.2019.00195. PMID: 31179251; PMCID: PMC6537603.

Gagnon H, Lunde CE, Wu Z, Novais EN, Borsook D, Sieberg CB. Exploring comorbidities in adolescent and young adults with hypermobile Ehlers-Danlos syndrome with and without a surgical history: A preliminary investigation. Children (Basel). 2023 Sep 16;10(9):1562. doi: 10.3390/children10091562. PMID: 37761523; PMCID: PMC10528958.

Peggs KJ, Nguyen H, Enayat D, Keller NR, Al-Hendy A, Raj SR. Gynecologic disorders and menstrual cycle lightheadedness in postural tachycardia syndrome. Int J Gynaecol Obstet. 2012 Sep;118(3):242–246. doi: 10.1016/j.ijgo.2012.04.014. Epub 2012 Jun 20. PMID: 22721633; PMCID: PMC3413773.

Belna S, Trotman G, G-L V. Endometriosis/pelvic pain syndromes and postural tachycardia syndrome: What is the association and treatment implications? Journal of Pediatric and Adolescent Gynecology. 2014 27(2):e59-e60 DOI:10.1016/j.jpag.2014.01.085.

Wang S, Farland LV, Gaskins AJ, Mortazavi J, Wang YX, Tamimi RM, Rich-Edwards JW, Zhang D, Terry KL, Chavarro JE, Missmer SA. Association of laparoscopically-confirmed endometriosis with long COVID-19: a prospective cohort study. Am J Obstet Gynecol. 2023 Jun; 228(6):714.e1–714.e13. doi: 10.1016/j.ajog.2023.03.030. Epub 2023 Mar 25. PMID: 36972892; PMCID: PMC10101545.

Vasilev S. Mast cell activation syndrome and endometriosis: A potential link for unexplained symptoms in women. Gynecologic Oncology Institute, Robotic Surgery, Integrative Healing. 2023;4 Mar.

Shigesi N, Kvaskoff M, Kirtley S, Feng Q, Fang H, Knight JC, Missmer SA, Rahmioglu N, Zondervan KT, Becker CM. The association between endometriosis and autoimmune diseases: A systematic review and meta-analysis. Hum Reprod Update. 2019 Jul 1;25(4):486–503. doi: 10.1093/humupd/dmz014. PMID: 31260048; PMCID: PMC6601386.

Chapter 5: Feeling Sick and Tired of Feeling Sick and Tired and Other Mental Health Impacts

Hambleton A, Pepin G, Le A, Maloney D, National Eating Disorder Research Consortium; Touyz S, Maguire S. Psychiatric and medical comorbidities of eating disorders: Findings from a rapid review of the literature. J Eat Disord. 2022 Sep 5;10(1):132. doi: 10.1186/s40337-022-00654-2. PMID: 36064606; PMCID: PMC9442924.

van Stein K, Schubert K, Ditzen B, Weise C. Understanding psychological symptoms of endometriosis from a research domain criteria perspective. J Clin Med. 2023 Jun 15;12(12):4056. doi: 10.3390/jcm12124056. PMID: 37373749; PMCID: PMC10299570.

Wang TM, Lee YL, Chung CH, Sun CA, Kang CY, Wu GJ, Chien WC. Association between endometriosis and mental disorders including psychiatric disorders, suicide, and all-cause mortality—A nationwide population-based cohort study in Taiwan. Int J Womens Health. 2023 Nov 28;15:1865–1882. doi: 10.2147/IJWH.S430252. PMID: 38046265; PMCID: PMC10693200.

Koller D, Pathak GA, Wendt FR, Tylee DS, Levey DF, Overstreet C, Gelernter J, Taylor HS, Polimanti R. Epidemiologic and genetic associations of endometriosis with depression, anxiety, and eating disorders. JAMA Netw Open. 2023 Jan 3;6(1):e2251214. doi: 10.1001/jamanetworkopen.2022.51214. PMID: 36652249; PMCID: PMC9856929.

Carbone MG, Campo G, Papaleo E, Marazziti D, Maremmani I. The importance of a multi-disciplinary approach to the endometriotic patients: The relationship between endometriosis and psychic vulnerability. J Clin Med. 2021 Apr 10;10(8):1616. doi: 10.3390/jcm10081616. PMID: 33920306; PMCID: PMC8069439.

Gao M, Koupil I, Sjöqvist H, Karlsson H, Lalitkumar S, Dalman C, Kosidou K. Psychiatric comorbidity among women with endometriosis: Nationwide cohort study in Sweden. American Journal of Obstetrics & Gynecology. 2020;223;3;415.e1–415.e16.

Chiuve SE, Kilpatrick RD, Hornstein MD, Petruski-Ivleva N, Wegrzyn LR, Dabrowski EC, Velentgas P, Snabes MC, Bateman BT. Chronic opioid use and complication risks in women with endometriosis: A cohort study in US administrative claims. Pharmacoepidemiol Drug Saf. 2021 Jun;30(6):787–796. doi: 10.1002/pds.5209. Epub 2021 Mar 16. PMID: 33611812; PMCID: PMC8251707.

Ward JH, Weir E, Allison C, Simon BC. Increased rates of chronic physical health conditions across all organ systems in autistic adolescents and adults. Molecular Autism 2023;14;35. https://doi.org/10.1186/s13229-023-00565-2.

Ishikura IA, Hachul H, Pires GN, Tufik S, Andersen ML. The relationship between insomnia and endometriosis. J Clin Sleep Med. 2020 Aug 15;16(8):1387–1388. doi: 10.5664/jcsm.8464. PMID: 32267223; PMCID: PMC7446064.

Soliman AM, Surrey E, Bonafede M, Nelson JK, Castelli-Haley J. Real-world evaluation of direct and indirect economic burden among endometriosis patients in the United States. Adv Ther. 2018 Mar;35(3):408–423. doi: 10.1007/s12325-018-0667-3. Epub 2018 Feb 15. PMID: 29450864; PMCID: PMC5859693.

Estes SJ, Soliman AM, Yang H, Wang J, Freimark J. A longitudinal assessment of the impact of endometriosis on patients' salary growth and risk of leaving the workforce. Adv Ther. 2020 May;37(5):2144–2158. doi: 10.1007/s12325-020-01280-7. Epub 2020 Mar 20. PMID: 32198641; PMCID: PMC7467493.

Kübler-Ross E. On death and dying. Routledge. 1973.

Endometriosis: Women "taking their own lives" due to lack of support. 2019, Oct. BBC News. https://bbc.com/news/uk-wales-49933866.

Zullo L, van Dyk IS, Ollen E, Ramos N, Asarnow J, Miranda J. Treatment recommendations and barriers to care for suicidal LGBTQ youth: A quality improvement study. Evid Based Pract Child Adolesc Ment Health. 2021;6(3):393–409. doi: 10.1080/23794925.2021.1950079. Epub 2021 Sep 24. PMID: 34901439; PMCID: PMC8659407.

Hsieh TYJ, Neuhausser W, Wei JCC, Modest AM. Associations between pre-pregnancy endometriosis and postpartum psychiatric disorders. Fertility and Sterility 2024;122(4), e24.

Grobman WA, Parker CB, Willinger M, Wing DA, Silver RM, Wapner RJ, Simhan HN, Parry S, Mercer BM, Haas DM, Peaceman AM, Hunter S, Wadhwa P, Elovitz MA, Foroud T, Saade G, Reddy UM. Eunice Kennedy Shriver National Institute of Child Health and Human Development Nulliparous Pregnancy Outcomes Study: Monitoring Mothers-to-Be (nuMoM2b) Network*. Racial Disparities in Adverse Pregnancy Outcomes and Psychosocial Stress. Obstet Gynecol. 2018 Feb;131(2):328–335. doi: 10.1097/AOG.0000000000002441. PMID: 29324613; PMCID: PMC5785441.

Greenfield M, Darwin Z. Trans and non-binary pregnancy, traumatic birth, and perinatal mental health: A scoping review. Int J Transgend Health. 2021 Nov 19;22(1–2):203–216. doi: 10.1080/26895269.2020.1841057. PMID: 34806082; PMCID: PMC8040683.

Hambleton A, Pepin G, Le A, Maloney D, National Eating Disorder Research Consortium; Touyz S, Maguire S. Psychiatric and medical comorbidities of eating disorders: Findings from a rapid review of the literature. J Eat Disord. 2022 Sep 5;10(1):132. doi: 10.1186/s40337-022-00654-2. PMID: 36064606; PMCID: PMC9442924.

Sperschneider ML, Hengartner MP, Kohl-Schwartz A, Geraedts K, Rauchfuss M, Woelfler MM, Haeberlin F, von Orelli S, Eberhard M, Maurer F, Imthurn B, Imesch P, Leeners B. Does endometriosis affect professional life? A matched case-control study in Switzerland, Germany and Austria. BMJ Open. 2019 Jan 9;9(1):e019570. doi: 10.1136/bmjopen-2017-019570. PMID: 30782670; PMCID: PMC6340011.

Missmer SA, Tu FF, Agarwal SK, Chapron C, Soliman AM, Chiuve S, Eichner S, Flores-Caldera I, Horne AW, Kimball AB, Laufer MR, Leyland N, Singh SS, Taylor HS, As-Sanie S. Impact of endometriosis on life-course potential: A narrative review. Int J Gen Med. 2021 Jan 7;14:9–25. doi: 10.2147/IJGM.S261139. PMID: 33442286; PMCID: PMC7800443.

Bird CM, Webb EK, Schramm AT, Torres L, Larson C, deRoon-Cassini TA. Racial discrimination is associated with acute posttraumatic stress symptoms and predicts future posttraumatic stress disorder symptom severity in trauma-exposed Black adults in the United States. J Trauma Stress. 2021 Oct;34(5):995–1004. doi: 10.1002/jts.22670. Epub 2021 Mar 14. PMID: 33715212; PMCID: PMC9123835.

Alonzo AA. The experience of chronic illness and post-traumatic stress disorder: The consequences of cumulative adversity. Social Science & Medicine 50;10,2000:1475–1484, ISSN 0277-9536, https://doi.org/10.1016/S0277-9536(99)00399-8.

Roozitalab S, Rahimzadeh M, Mirmajidi SR, Ataee M, Esmaelzadeh Saeieh S. The relationship between infertility, stress, and quality of life with posttraumatic stress disorder in infertile women. J Reprod Infertil. 2021 Oct–Dec;22(4):282–288. doi: 10.18502/jri.v22i4.7654. PMID: 34987990; PMCID: PMC8669410.

Ugwumadu L, Chakrabarti R, Williams-Brown E, Rendle K, Swift I, Babbin J, Allen-Coward H, Ofuasia E. The role of the multidisciplinary team in the management of deep infiltrating endometriosis. Gynecol Surg 2017 14;15. https://doi.org/10.1186/s10397-017-1018-0

Dong B, Wu CL, Sheng Yl, Wu B, Guan-Chao Y, Ha-Fei L, Shi-Hao L, Han L, Qi Y. Catamenial pneumothorax with bubbling up on the diaphragmatic defects: A case report. BMC Women's Health 2021;21;167. https://doi.org/10.1186/s12905-021-01318-0.

Wolthuis AM, Meuleman C, Tomassetti C, D'Hooghe T, de Buck van Overstraeten A, D'Hoore A. Bowel endometriosis: Colorectal surgeon's perspective in a multidisciplinary surgical team. World J Gastroenterol. 2014 Nov 14;20(42):15616–15623. doi: 10.3748/wjg.v20.i42.15616. PMID: 25400445; PMCID: PMC4229526.

Nezhat C, Paka C, Gomaa M, Schipper E. Silent loss of kidney secondary to ureteral endometriosis. JSLS. 2012 Jul–Sep;16(3):451–455. doi: 10.4293/108680812X13462882736213. PMID: 23318072; PMCID: PMC3535807.

Bontempo AC, Mikesell L. Patient perceptions of misdiagnosis of endometriosis: Results from an online national survey. Diagnosis (Berl). 2020 May 26;7(2):97–106. doi: 10.1515/dx-2019-0020. PMID: 32007945.

Chapter 6: From Harm to Hope

United Nations Children's Fund & World Health Organization. Progress on household drinking water, sanitation and hygiene 2000–2022: Special focus on gender. World Health Organization. 2024.

Unicef. https://data.unicef.org/resources/sofi-2023/ 2023 July.

National Low Income Housing Coalition. https://nlihc.org/resource/hud-releases-2023-annual-homeless-assessment-report 2023 Dec.

Jaafar H, Ismail SY, Azzeri A. Period poverty: A neglected public health issue. Korean J Fam Med. 2023 Jul;44(4):183–188. doi: 10.4082/kjfm.22.0206. Epub 2023 May 16. PMID: 37189262; PMCID: PMC10372806.

Gupta J, Cardoso L, Kanselaar S, Scolese AM, Hamidaddin A, Pollack AZ, Earnshaw VA. Life disruptions, symptoms suggestive of endometriosis, and anticipated stigma among college students in the United States. Womens Health Rep. 2021;2(1):633–642. doi:10.1089/whr.2021.0072.

Mandeville J, Earnshaw VA, Zhang C, Cardoso LF, Gupta J. Associations between stigma and depression among college-attending women with endometriosis symptoms. Journal of American College Health, 2014;73(3);989–999. https://doi.org/10.1080/07448481.2024.2422319.

González-Echevarría AM, Rosario E, Acevedo S, Flores I. Impact of coping strategies on quality of life of adolescents and young women with endometriosis. J Psychosom Obstet Gynaecol. 2019;40(2):138–145. doi:10.1080/0167482X.2018.1450384.

Center for Substance Abuse Treatment (US). Trauma-informed care in behavioral health services. Rockville (MD): Substance Abuse and Mental Health Services Administration (US); 2014. (Treatment Improvement Protocol (TIP) Series, No. 57.) Chapter 1, Trauma-Informed Care: A Sociocultural Perspective. https://www.ncbi.nlm.nih.gov/books/NBK207195/.

Banja JD. Medical errors and medical narcissism. Jones & Bartlett Learning 2024.

Trayer J, Rowbotham NJ, Boyle RJ, Smyth AR. Industry influence in healthcare harms patients: Myth or maxim? Breathe (Sheff). 2022 Jun;18(2):220010. doi: 10.1183/20734735.0010-2022. Epub 2022 Jul 12. PMID: 36337122; PMCID: PMC9584590.

Hunter M (ed.). Women's health and corporate marketing our bodies, their business. Under the influence: Pharmaceutical relationships & their impact on endometriosis care. Heather Guidone 2025, chapter 4.

Kirk UB, Bank-Mikkelsen AS, Rytter D, Hartwell D, Marschall H, Nyegaard M, Seyer-Hansen M, Ejgaard Hansen K. Understanding endometriosis underfunding and its detrimental impact on awareness and research. npj Womens Health 2024;2;45. https://doi.org/10.1038/s44294-024-00048-6.

Index

ablation technique, 22–23
abuse, 126–127, 132–133, 140
   gaslighting, 139
academic institutions, 168, 170–171
acceptance, 105, 176–177
accessibility to treatment, 27–28
ACESSA procedure, 71
Addison's disease, 88–89
adenomyosis, 66–68
advocacy, 28–29, 166, 167, 187–188
   initiatives, 168–169
   self-advocacy, 173–174, 177–178
age of diagnosis, 8–11
anorexia nervosa, 114–115
anxiety, 94–99
   diagnosis, 99–101
attention-deficit/hyperactivity disorder (ADHD), 93
autism, 93
autoimmune disorders, 86–90
autoimmune thyroid disorder, 89
autonomic nervous system, 81–83
avoidant restrictive food intake disorder (ARFID), 115–116

babies, endometriosis in, 9
binge eating disorder, 115
biochemical pregnancy, 50
BIPOC communities, 29, 45, 49, 51
   abuse, 126
   risk of fibroids, 70
blood tests, 14
boundaries, 132–133, 144, 180–181
bowel endometriosis, 14, 17
bulimia nervosa, 115

caregiving, 147
celiac disease, 87–88
childhood trauma, 100
children (*see also* teenagers)
   endometriosis in, 9
   impact of parental illness on, 147
   parental figures, 135–137

chronic fatigue syndrome (CFS), 77–78
combined hormonal contraceptives, 18
comorbidities, 8, 51, 65–90
competency, 129–130, 144
COVID-19, Long COVID, 83–84
Crohn's disease, 88
cystoscopy, 73

denial, 130–131
depression
   after childbirth, 111–112
   diagnosis, 105–106
despair, 132, 145
diagnosis
   age of, 8–11
   difficulties, 11–12
   suspected, 13–15
diet, 114
dignity, 129, 144
dyspareunia, 39

eating disorders, 112–117
ectopic pregnancy, 31, 50–51
educating yourself, 177
education for healthcare providers, 185–186
embolization, 71
emotional needs, 127–128, 140–143, 161–163
emotions, 140
   in teenagers, 152
empathy, 141
employment, 126, 167–168
   interventions, 171–172
endometriosis, definition, 1–2
environmental needs, 127
ethics, 187–188
examinations, pain during, 44–45
excision surgery, 12–13, 21–22, 48, 53

female bladder pain syndrome (FBPS), 71–73
feminism, 37
fertility *see* infertility
fertility treatment, pain during, 44–45
fibroids, 68–71
fibromyalgia syndrome, 76–77
financial impact of infertility, 46
flexibility, 181–183
   from friends and family, 142

gaslighting, 139
genetic links, 6, 134
GnRH agonists, 19–20
GnRH antagonists, 20
goals, 131–132
government policies, 167, 169–170
grief, 102–105, 181–182
gynecological oncologists, 25–26

Hashimoto's disease, 66, 89
healthcare insecurity, 126
healthcare providers, 10 (*see also* medical industrial complex (MIC))
   approaches to medical care, 185–188
   dismissive attitudes, 28–29, 33–37, 47, 118
   education, 185–186
   expert endometriosis surgeons, 21–22, 48, 53
   gynecological oncologists, 25–26
   ignorance, 24–25, 134–135
   maternal fetal medicine specialists, 53, 55
   narcissism, 161–163
   OB/GYNs, 22–23, 26, 55
   pelvic floor therapists, 23, 41, 58
   reimbursement, 27–28
   reproductive endocrinologists (REIs), 47–48, 53
   reproductive immunologists, 53
   safety needs, 159–161
   trust in, 134–135
hope, 174, 182
hormonal treatments, 4
   combined hormonal contraceptives, 18
   for diagnosis, 14–15
   hormone replacement therapy (HRT), 60–61, 62
   progesterone and progestins, 19
hypermobile Ehlers-Danlos Syndrome (hEDS), 79–81
hysterectomy, 68, 70
hysteria, 34

imaging tests, 13–14
inclusivity, 142
independence, 129
infertility, 31, 42–49
inflammatory bowel disease, 88
initiatives, 168–169
institutional awareness, 165–172
interstitial cystitis (IC), 71–73
interventions, 169–172, 186–187
IVF treatment, 46–47

kidneys, 14

laparoscopic surgery, 12, 70–71
legislation, 30–31
   on abortion rights in the US, 52
   on IVF treatments, 46–47
LGBTQIA+ community, 29–30, 46, 49
   abuse, 126
   mental health, 108
limitations, 131–132
Long COVID, 83–84
loss, feelings of, 102–105
lungs, 14

Maslow's hierarchy of needs, 123–133, 138–146
   applicable to the MIC, 159–165
Mast Cell Activation Syndrome (MCAS), 85–86
maternal fetal medicine specialists, 53, 55
media, inaccuracies, 166–167
medical abuse, 126–127
medical harm, 187–188
medical imaging, 13–14
medical industrial complex (MIC), 153–159
   and hierarchy of needs, 159–165
medical narcissism, 161–163

medical trauma, 118–122
medications, 17–20
  side effects, 40
menopause, 10–11, 58–63
mental health, 25, 91–122
  affected by sexual dysfunction, 40, 41
  and infertility, 45
  and pregnancy complications, 57–58
  and pregnancy loss, 52, 54
  in teenagers, 150–151
miscarriage, 31, 49–50, 51–52
misogyny, 29, 36
morcellation, 71
multidisciplinary approach to treatment, 17–31, 49
  for pregnancy loss, 54
multiple sclerosis (MS), 88
myalgic encephalomyelitis (ME), 77–78
myomectomy, 70–71
myths about endometriosis, 3–6

narcissism, 161–163
needs, 123–133, 123–146, 138–146
  applicable to the MIC, 159–165
  self-advocacy, 174–175
  values needed, 176–183
neurodivergence, 93
NSAIDs, 18

OB/GYNs, 22–23, 26, 55
orthorexia, 116
other specified feeding or eating disorder (OSFED), 116

pain management, 36
parental figures, 135–137
patient advocacy, 28–29
patriarchy, 33–35, 36, 163–164
peer support groups, 178
pelvic floor therapists, 23, 41, 58
pelvic pain, 40
perimenopause, 58–63
physiological needs, 124–125, 138, 159
placenta previa, 57
placental abruption, 57

pneumothorax, 14
politicians, 30–31
polycystic ovary syndrome (PCOS), 74–75
postpartum depression, 111–112
post-traumatic stress disorder (PTSD), 118–122
Postural Orthostatic Tachycardia Syndrome (POTS), 81–83
preeclampsia, 56–57
pregnancy, 31
  complications, 54–58
  loss, 31, 49–54, 92
  pain during, 56
premenstrual dysphoric disorder (PMDD), 109, 110
premenstrual exacerbation (PME), 110–111
premenstrual syndrome (PMS), 109–110
presacral neurectomy, 68
progesterone and progestins, 19

racism, 29, 45, 51, 126
radical acceptance, 176–177
rectal nodules, 14
reframing, 179–180
relationships, 127–128
  affected by sexual dysfunction, 40–42
  boundaries in, 132–133, 144
  friends and family, 133–146
  impact of illness on, 146–147
  unhealthy, 172–173
reproductive endocrinologists (REIs), 47–48, 53
reproductive immunologists, 53
rheumatoid arthritis, 87

safety needs, 125–127, 138–140, 159–161
self-actualization needs, 130–131, 145–146, 164–165
self-advocacy, 173–174, 177–178
self-awareness, 180
self-criticism, 100–101, 131, 179–180
self-esteem, 128–130, 143–144, 163–164
self-love, 177

self-worth, 128–129
sexual abuse, 42
sexual dysfunction, 38–42
sexual intercourse, 33
sexual trauma, 5
shame, feelings of, 35–36
Sjogren's disease, 89
social media, 63
social needs, 127–128, 140–143, 161–163
societal interventions, 169
standards of care, 26
stigma, 30, 35–36
 of sexual dysfunction, 40–41
stillbirth, 50
subspecialties, 25–26
suicidal thoughts, 108–109
support, 30
 from friends and family, 133–146
 for infertility, 47
 peer support groups, 49, 178
 for perimenopause and menopause, 62–63
 for pregnancy complications, 58
 for pregnancy loss, 52–53
 team approach, 133–134, 176–183
surgery, 21
 anxiety about, 98–99
 laparoscopic, 12
 medical trauma from, 121
 surgical excision, 12–13, 21–22, 48, 53
suspected diagnosis, 13–15
symptoms of endometriosis, 6–8

systemic lupus erythematosus (SLE), 87
systems affected by endometriosis, 4

team approach, 133–134, 176–183
teenagers
 endometriosis in, 8–9, 147–152
 polycystic ovary syndrome (PCOS) in, 75
tests for endometriosis, 13–15
thoracic endometriosis, 14
trauma
 childhood, 100
 medical, 118–122
treatment, 4
 accessibility, 27–28
 for female bladder pain syndrome (FBPS), 73
 for fibroids, 70–71
 merry-go-round, 106–108
 multidisciplinary approach, 17–31, 49, 54

ulcerative colitis, 88
ultrasound scans, 13–14
uncertainty, 97–98
ureteral endometriosis, 14
uterine anomalies, 56, 57
uterine artery embolization, 71
uterine fibroids, 68–71
uterus, 66–68

weight changes, 112–113
workplace, 126, 167–168
 interventions, 171–172

About the author

Casey Berna has a Master's of Social Work from Fordham University and is a licensed clinical social worker. She currently maintains her own private practice where she specializes in supporting patients dealing with stress, anxiety, grief, and medical trauma in the endometriosis, infertility, pregnancy loss and chronic illness communities.

As a long-standing patient advocate, Casey has collaborated with Project Endo, The Endometriosis Research Center, The Endometriosis Summit, The Endometriosis Coalition, The Sister-Girl Foundation, and the Latina Endometriosis League of America to improve access to care while calling attention to the mental health impact of endometriosis and infertility. She has also had the pleasure of working with other nonprofits in the community, such as Gynoqueer, Extrapelvic Not Rare, and received EndoBlack, Inc.'s, Outstanding Ally award at their inaugural gala. Her documentary, "Endotruths: Impact of Endometriosis and Infertility on Mental Health," was featured in the Unmentionables Film Festival in Harlem, New York.

Join the Sheldon Press community today, sign up for our newsletter!

- Select a **FREE eBook** or extract to read upon joining

- Keep up with our latest publishing and exciting author news

- Be the first to hear about book prize draws, free extracts, and upcoming author events

Simply scan the QR code below or head to www.sheldonpress.co.uk/newsletter to sign up.

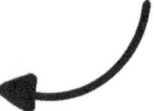